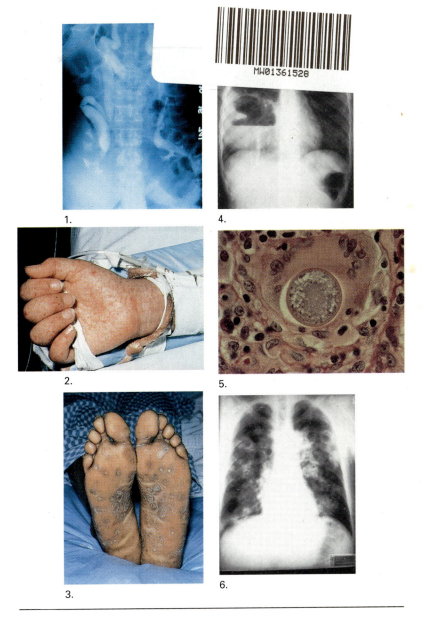

Color Plate 1. Renal tuberculosis: distorted, "sausage-link" ureters are the result of focal ureteral scarring.

Color Plate 2. Rocky Mountain Spotted Fever with diffuse petechial eruption.

Color Plate 3. Secondary syphilis: papular eruption includes palms and soles.

Color Plate 4. Lung abscess (*Klebsiella pneumoniae*).

Color Plate 5. Coccidioidomycosis: Spherule within giant cell in skin biopsy of patient with disseminated infection.

Color Plate 6. Nocardiosis: multiple cavitating lesions in chest x-ray of patient treated with corticosteriods for idiopathic thrombocytopenic purpura.

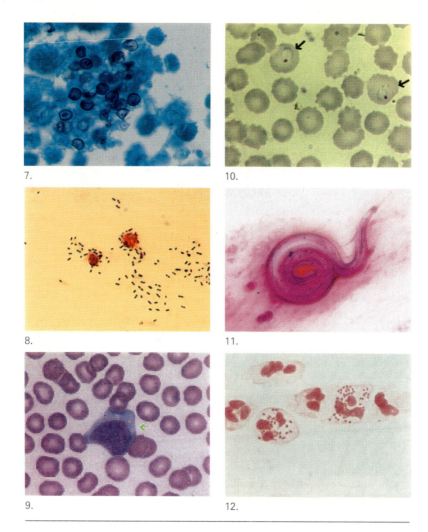

Color Plate 7. *Pneumocystis carinii* pneumonia (PCP) in patient with AIDS. (Gomori methenamine silver stain.)

Color Plate 8. Pneumococcal meningitis. Gram stain of cerebrospinal fluid.

Color Plate 9. Atypical lymphocyte in patient with infectious mononucleosis. Cytoplasm is "molded" by contiguous erythrocytes.

Color Plate 10. Malaria (*P. vivax*). Note ring trophozoites (arrows) in young erythrocytes, which are larger and paler than the other (older) erythrocytes.

Color Plate 11. Strongyloidiasis. Larval forms may be found in stool or, as with this patient with hyperinfection syndrome, in the sputum.

Color Plate 12. Gonococcal urethritis. Gram stain shows polymorphonuclear leukocytes with intracytoplasmic Gram-negative diplococci.

DIFFERENTIAL DIAGNOSIS OF INFECTIOUS DISEASES

DIFFERENTIAL DIAGNOSIS OF INFECTIOUS DISEASES

David Schlossberg, MD
Director, Department of Medicine
Episcopal Hospital
Professor of Medicine
The Medical College of Pennsylvania and Hahnemann University
Philadelphia, Pennsylvania

Jonas A. Shulman, MD
Professor of Medicine
Associate Dean for Medical Education and Student Affairs
Emory University School of Medicine
Atlanta, Georgia

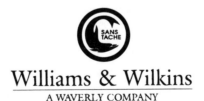

Williams & Wilkins
A WAVERLY COMPANY

BALTIMORE • PHILADELPHIA • LONDON • PARIS • BANGKOK
BUENOS AIRES • HONG KONG • MUNICH • SYDNEY • TOKYO • WROCLAW
1996

Editor: Jonathan W. Pine, Jr.
Managing Editor: Molly L. Mullen
Production Coordinator: Marette D. Magargle-Smith
Copy Editor: Alice Lium
Designer: Julie Burris
Illustration Planner: Ray Lowman
Cover Designer: Julie Burris
Typesetter: Maryland Composition
Printer: Victor Graphics
Binder: Victor Graphics

351 West Camden Street
Baltimore, Maryland 21201-2436 USA

Rose Tree Corporate Center
1400 North Providence Road
Building II, Suite 5025
Media, Pennsylvania 19063-2043 USA

Copyright © 1996 Williams & Wilkins

Some of the material in this book was previously published in *Handbook for Differential Diagnosis of Infectious Diseases,* by Jonas A. Shulman and David Schlossberg. Copyright 1980 by Appleton-Century-Crofts, a Publishing Division of Prentice-Hall, Inc., New York, New York.

All rights reserved. This book is protected by copyright. No part of this book may be reproduced in any form or by any means, including photocopying, or utilized by any information storage and retrieval system without written permission from the copyright owner.

Accurate indications, adverse reactions and dosage schedules for drugs are provided in this book, but it is possible that they may change. The reader is urged to review the package information data of the manufacturers of the medications mentioned.

Printed in the United States of America

First Edition,

Library of Congress Cataloging-in-Publication Data

Schlossberg, David.
   Differential diagnosis of infectious diseases / David Schlossberg, Jonas A. Shulman.
     p. cm.
   Some of the material in this book was previously published in
Handbook for differential diagnosis of infectious diseases, by Jonas
A. Shulman and David Schlossberg. c1980—T.p. verso.
   Includes bibliographical references and index.
   ISBN 0-683-07659-0
   1. Communicable diseases—Diagnosis. 2. Diagnosis, Differential.
I. Shulman, Jonas A., 1936–   . II. Shulman, Jonas A., 1936–.
Handbook for differential diagnosis of infectious diseases.
III. Title.
   [DNLM: 1. Communicable Diseases—diagnosis. 2. Diagnosis,
Differential.   WC 100 S345d 1996]
RC112.S33 1996
616.9'0475—dc20
DNLM/DLC
for Library of Congress   95-4784
                                                                                        CIP

The publishers have made every effort to trace the copyright holders for borrowed material. If they have inadvertently overlooked any, they will be pleased to make the necessary arrangements at the first opportunity.

96 97 98 99
1 2 3 4 5 6 7 8 9 10

Reprints of chapters may be purchased from Williams & Wilkins in quantities of 100 or more. Call Isabella Wise, Special Sales Department, (800) 358-3583.

We dedicate this volume to our many students and
house staff, who continue to challenge and inspire us.

הרבה למדתי מרבותי ומחביריי יותר מרבותי ומתלמידי יותר מכולן

"Much have I learned from my teachers,
and from my colleagues even more than my teachers,
and from my students the most of all."

—*Babylonian Talmud, Tractate Ta'anit.*

PREFACE

AIDS, Lyme disease, *Clostridium difficile*, Parvovirus, and *Chlamydia pneumoniae* are only a fraction of the new diseases that have appeared since we published an earlier version of this book 15 years ago. In addition, etiologies for older diseases like Whipple's disease and cat scratch disease have finally been established. It has been reassuring to some and surprising to others that the specialty of infectious diseases continues to change so rapidly.

The expansion challenges even further the clinician's ability to form a differential diagnosis. As with the first book, our goal with this much revised and updated version is to orient the evaluation of patients with a classic clinical presentation, organizing the differential diagnosis in both textual and chart form, and providing additional clinically pertinent data regarding lab diagnosis, transmission of infection, and therapy. In general, the orientation is toward infectious disease entities seen in the U.S.A.

This text complements, but does not replace, the more detailed texts available on the subject of infectious disease. However, it does help initiate and facilitate the evaluation of patients who have signs and symptoms that may suggest a large variety of infectious diagnoses.

Some technologic aspects of infectious disease diagnosis are evolving rapidly. For example, molecular biological techniques for diagnosis are being developed for many pathogens. Current literature must be constantly reviewed to remain abreast of these and other diagnostic and therapeutic advances; nevertheless, the basic clinical approach in this text should help in the clinical organization of an increasingly complex and challenging discipline.

We gratefully acknowledge the support for our color figures from Bristol-Myers, Dupont, Hoechst, Janssen, Merck, Pfizer, and Wyeth-Ayerst.

CONTENTS

Preface vii
Chapter 1. Fever 1
Chapter 2. Acute Pneumonitis 13
Chapter 3. Cerebrospinal Fluid Pleocytosis 53
Chapter 4. Bacteriuria and Pyuria 87
Chapter 5. Diarrhea 113
Chapter 6. Rash 133
Chapter 7. Monoarthritis 163
Chapter 8. Polyarthritis 171
Chapter 9. Jaundice 195
Chapter 10. Splenomegaly 213
Chapter 11. Localized and Generalized Lymphadenopathy 227
Chapter 12. The Compromised Host 261
Chapter 13. AIDS 279

Chapter 14. Hematologic Changes Associated With Infection 301

Chapter 15. Sources and Transmission of Infectious Diseases Other Than Person-to-Person-Spread 307

Recommended Reading 313

Index 319

1

FEVER

Many disease states may cause a rise in body temperature, including infection, neoplastic disease, and autoimmune disorders. Current thinking suggests that the final common pathway in the production of fever is probably the production of endogenous pyrogens (interleukein 1, tumor necrosis factor, interferon alpha and possibly others) from polymorphonuclear leukocytes (PMLs), monocytes, macrophages and other tissues during the process of inflammation. These pyrogens in turn act on the hypothalamus with resultant release of arachidonic acid. Arachidonic acid is metabolized to prostaglandins and other substances which then elevate the hypothalamic thermostat.

Before considering pathogenic states that cause fever, it is important to understand the normal variation in human body temperature. First, although a temperature of 98.6 F is considered normal, many patients' highest daily temperature may range from 97 to 99.6 F. In addition to the variability in the peak temperatures among patients, there is also a variation of about one degree Fahrenheit in each individual every day. The highest daily temperature usually occurs in the late afternoon or early evening, and the nadir is at about 4:00 A.M. This variation is exaggerated with fever, but may be reversed in old age, in miliary tuberculosis, and by salicylate administration. The rectal temperature is usually about one degree higher than the oral, which in turn is one degree higher than the axillary temperature. Outside the range of this normal variation, there are several physiologic states that can cause fever. These include digestion, exercise, ovulation, pregnancy, warm environment, and emotion.

Of the pathologic causes of fever, infection is both the most frequent and most important to diagnose early, since specific treatment may be indicated. However, before discussing specific etiologies of fever, several variations in the ability of the host to respond to tissue injury or infection with fever must be considered. For example, the very young may have an exaggerated febrile response to infection. Infants often first announce infection by a febrile convulsion, which results from a rapid and very pronounced rise in temperature. Although fevers of 105 to 107 F are not terribly uncommon in the young, adults rarely have extreme elevation in temperature (107 to 108 F) except with heat stroke, cerebral infarction, or the postoperative complication of malignant hyperpyrexia secondary to administration of certain muscle relaxants and anesthetics. On the other hand, elderly patients tend to have a diminished temperature response to infection, but when febrile they may become disoriented.

FEVER PATTERNS

Classically, observers have described four patterns of fever in an attempt to associate specific diseases with the type of fever they cause. These four patterns are (a) intermittent (high spikes with return to normal), (b) remittent (like intermittent, but the temperature never returns to normal), (c) sustained (like remittent, but with less marked swings of temperature), and (d) relapsing (several days of fever alternating with periods of normal temperature). Unfortunately, this categorization is not terribly helpful. There are many exceptions to these typical patterns and many factors affect the temperature response and may change the fever pattern in the individual patient. For example, although a history of recurrent chills and fever suggests a disease that causes extreme swings of temperature, if the patient has been taking salicylates, his chills may result from the rapid defervescence caused by antipyretic administration.

Although the fever pattern is generally not helpful in differential diagnosis, a few patterns do suggest specific diseases. For example, typhoid fever classically manifests a sustained temperature elevation, while fever from an abscess is typically remittent. A relapsing fever is particularly helpful, since it may indicate malaria, rat-bite fever, cholangitis, or infection with *Borrelia recurrentis*. Important noninfectious causes of relapsing fever include Hodgkin's disease and intermittent obstruction of the common bile duct by stone or by a carcinoma.

In some diseases only two episodes of fever occur, separated by a brief afebrile interval. This type of fever pattern suggests leptospirosis, Colorado tick fever, lymphocytic choriomeningitis, and dengue.

The most specific fever pattern is the double quotidian fever, with two daily spikes. Miliary tuberculosis, gonococcal or meningococcal endocarditis, kala-azar, Q fever, and juvenile rheumatoid arthritis should be considered when this occurs. However, there are limits to the specificity of a temperature curve, and a more useful classification of fever is (1) short term, (2) long term, and (3) hospital acquired (Table 1.1).

FEVER IN NONHOSPITALIZED PATIENTS

Those brief fevers (less than one week) occurring in the nonhospitalized population are usually caused by self-limited viral illnesses. The most common nonviral causes of short-term fever are bacterial infection of the throat, ear, paranasal sinuses, bronchi, or urinary tract.

Patients who remain febrile for more than one to two weeks require more intensive investigation. It is this group that presents with what has been conveniently called "fever of undetermined origin," or FUO.

Occasionally there is reason to doubt the veracity of a patient's illness, and one way of simulating organic illness is to present the physician with a temperature elevation that the patient himself has contrived. There are some physiologic clues to this "factitious fever." These include a temperature greater than 106 F, which is

4 DIFFERENTIAL DIAGNOSIS OF INFECTIOUS DISEASES

TABLE 1.1. THE PATIENT WITH FEVER

A. Short term
   1. Viral
   2. Bacterial infection of ear, throat, nasal sinuses, lungs, urinary tract

B. Long term
   1. Infection
      a. Systemic (tuberculosis, subacute bacterial endocarditis)
      b. Local (abscesses in liver, abdomen, GU tract)
   2. Tumors (lymphoma, leukemia, hypernephroma, disseminated carcinoma)
   3. Collagen-vascular disease
   4. Hypersensitivity states
   5. Miscellaneous (granulomatous disease, inflammatory bowel disease, pulmonary emboli, and many less frequent disorders)

C. Hospital acquired
   1. Normal host
      a. Infection at site of surgery
      b. Drug fever
      c. Respiratory complication (atelectasis, emboli, pneumonia)
      d. Urinary tract infection
      e. Phlebitis
      f. Inadequate drainage of fluid
   2. Compromised host
      a. Causes of fever in the normal host still the most frequent (see above)
      b. Also consider infection with opportunistic organisms
      c. Possible tumor-related fever

extremely rare in adults, a rapid fall in temperature without a concomitant diaphoresis, a lack of diurnal variation in the temperature curve, a lack of a rise in heart and respiratory rate with the fever, and a disparity between the measured rectal temperature and the temperature of a freshly voided urine sample. (At times there are exceptions to the usual rise in heart rate with fever, notably in certain infections, e.g., typhoid fever, mycoplasmal pneumonia, and psittacosis.) Factitious fever should be considered especially in individuals involved in health care fields.

Infection is a very important cause of treatable FUOs. A useful categorization of infectious etiologies of FUOs divides the causes into a systemic and a localized group of illnesses. The most frequent systemic diseases responsible for FUO are tuberculosis (usually miliary) and subacute bacterial endocarditis (SBE). Miliary tuberculosis need not produce a positive skin test, and the chest x-ray may lack a miliary pattern on admission to the hospital and may, in fact, even remain normal. Diagnosis is most often made by biopsy and culture of liver and marrow. SBE may be similarly difficult to detect. Blood cultures are negative in 15% of cases, and patients have been described without murmurs. Also, the classical peripheral stigmata (Osler's nodes, Janeway spots, splinter hemorrhages, splenomegaly, and Roth spots) are now rarely seen. Some of the less common systemic infections causing FUOs seen in this country are brucellosis, toxoplasmosis, cytomegalovirus (CMV) infection, chronic meningococcemia, and salmonellosis. Other than the hepatitis viruses, CMV, and Epstein-Barr virus (EBV), viral disease is a rare cause of prolonged febrile illness.

Localized infections that cause FUO are frequently located in clinically silent areas such as the abdomen and pelvis, rendering their detection difficult. In the abdomen, an obscure abscess is often found in the right upper quadrant either within the liver or in the subphrenic or subhepatic location. Intermittent obstruction of the biliary tree may produce cholangitis with "Charcot's intermittent biliary fever." The other intra-abdominal location that is important to investigate is the retroperitoneal space, where renal carbuncle, perinephric abscess, pyelonephritis with obstruction, and psoas abscess may present as obscure causes of fever. The female pelvis is another area to investigate when searching for a silent focus of infection.

About one-third of prolonged FUO will be caused by infection. An additional 20 to 40% will be caused by collagen vascular diseases such as systemic lupus erythematosus (SLE), rheumatoid arthritis, polyarthritis, polymyalgia rheumatica, rheumatic fever, and mixed collagen disease processes. The majority of the remaining causes of prolonged FUO are tumors, especially of the hematologic variety such as acute leukemias and lymphomas. Metastatic solid tumors, e.g., hypernephroma, hepatoma, carcinoma of the ampulla of Vater, bowel adenocarcinomas, at times present with fever as a major finding. Some localized tumors produce fever by causing infection in obstructed areas, e.g., a bronchogenic carcinoma with a pneumonitis in the obstructed lung segment, but these are usually readily diagnosed on routine examinations.

A variety of noninfectious causes of FUO account for most of the remaining etiologies and include pulmonary emboli, sarcoidosis, relapsing panniculitis (Weber-Christian disease), drug fever, familial Mediterranean fever, periodic fever, hyperthyroidism, Addison's disease, inflammatory bowel disease, and nonspecific granulomatous disease of the liver.

Initial laboratory procedures in the evaluation of a patient with FUO include routine complete blood count, serologic tests for syphilis, sedimentation rate, chest x-ray, liver function tests, urine analysis, stool for occult blood, stool and urine cultures, three to six sets of blood cultures, and sonography of the abdomen and pelvis. Skin tests for tuberculosis and checks for anergy (Candida, trichophyton, and streptokinase-streptodornase skin tests) are indicated (Table 1.2).

Depending on the clinical clues, one would next go to such studies as antinuclear antibody, rheumatoid factor, febrile agglutinins for salmonella and brucella and the mono-spot test. A tube of serum for other serologies should be frozen so more studies can be done if other diagnoses are suggested. A lumbar puncture (LP) should be performed if even the slightest indications exist such as backache, headache, or minimal mental changes. If no clues are forthcoming, the next group of procedures would involve intravenous pyelography and gall bladder studies, liver scan, and bone marrow with biopsy and culture followed by complete radiographic bowel studies.

The workup of FUO becomes increasingly invasive as the etiology remains obscure (Table 1.2). Often the patient will manifest a pathologic skin lesion or enlarged lymph node that is accessible to biopsy. However, the most productive biopsy sites are the liver and bone marrow. Liver biopsy often establishes a diagnosis even when only minimal derangement of liver function tests are present. Appropriate smears and cultures should be performed on biopsy specimens and body fluids and should include a workup to detect aerobes, anaerobes, tubercle bacilli, and fungi.

CT or MRI are useful in delineating abscesses or tumors in such organs as liver, pancreas and bone. Angiography, though more invasive, frequently may outline an abscess or tumor or show the characteristic vascular changes seen in thrombotic disease or certain types of vasculitis, e.g., polyarteritis nodosa.

When the cause of FUO remains obscure, there is often consideration of a therapeutic trial, which usually involves administration of antibiotics, antituberculous agents, heparin (for pulmonary emboli), or discontinuation of current medications for presumed drug fever. Such a trial yields the most information when the therapy used is highly specific; for example, a response to antituberculous therapy with isoniazid and ethambutol is more helpful than a response to antituberculous therapy with a regimen that includes streptomycin or rifampin because of the broad antibacterial spectrum of the latter two agents.

Finally, laparotomy may on occasion establish the diagnosis, but this is an extreme measure and should be employed only after careful deliberation. It is most helpful in finding small abscesses, especially in the right upper quadrant and in the pelvis.

With the increasing availability of international travel, the clinician is often faced with an FUO in a patient who has traveled abroad. This important history adds an additional list of diagnostic possibilities. The list might include, depending on the specific country visited, malaria, typhoid fever, hepatitis A and E, rickettsial and arbovirus infection, amebic liver abscess, typanosomiasis, leishmaniasis, brucellosis and melioidosis.

FEVER IN HOSPITALIZED PATIENTS

When fever is acquired by hospitalized patients, one must consider the following group of causes: (1) postoperative complications, e.g., wound infection or abscess; (2) drug fever; (3) respiratory complications, including pneumonia, atelectasis, and pulmonary embolus; (4) urinary tract infection; (5) phlebitis, especially around IV sites; and (6) inadequate drainage of fluid (e.g., pleural fluid) whether infected or sterile. A temperature elevation of one to two degrees is sometimes seen for a brief period (24 to 48 hours) in patients following admission to the hospital for diseases not usually accompanied by fever. This may be an example of so-called "psychogenic fever."

Drug fever is surprisingly common in hospitalized patients. All drugs should be considered potential culprits, with the possible exceptions of digitalis preparations. Clues to drug fever include pulse-temperature dissociation, eosinophilia, atypical lymphocytosis and rash, but frequently these signs are missing, and the patient has fever only.

When fever develops in the hospitalized patient who is immunosuppressed, either because of an underlying disease (e.g., cancer) or because of the effects of administration of immunosuppressive or antibiotic therapy, careful evaluation for infection is indicated. Fever in this group of patients is usually due to the same causes outlined above for the "normal" hospitalized population, but in addition, the immunosuppressed group is prone to infection with unusual organisms, especially *Candida, Aspergillus, Phycomycetes*, varicella-zoster, CMV, *Pneumocystis, Toxoplasma, Listeria, Legionella*, and *Nocardia*.

Some of these opportunistic agents may produce infections in sites from which clinical specimens are easily obtained. For example, spinal fluid, blood, and urine can be examined and cultured with ease. However, when the lung is involved, though sputum should be obtained, it is not always diagnostic. Therefore, in such situations bronchoscopy with biopsy, open-lung biopsy or needle aspiration may be necessary to establish the diagnosis, e.g., *Pneumocystis carinii* pneumonia.

When a patient with fever is acutely ill, empiric antibiotic therapy should be instituted, pending results of cultures. This therapy must be directed against the most likely site-specific pathogens, e.g., streptococci, anaerobes and Gram-negative enteric bacilli for bowel origin, enterococcus and Gram negative bacilli for genitourinary sepsis, etc. It is important to remember that some patients with septicemia, especially at extremes of age, will lack cardinal signs of infection such as leukocytosis and fever, or may have nonspecific signs of sepsis, such as unexplained hypotension, hypothermia, hypoglycemia, decreased urinary output or confusion.

Fever should be considered as possibly infectious in origin, requiring careful evaluation for treatable etiologies, although at times the fever may be related to the basic underlying disease process such as Hodgkin's disease or leukemia or to the chemotherapy such as bleomycin. When it is due to the tumor, fever often responds to treatment with Naprosen, whereas fever from infection and vasculitis does not.

TABLE 1.2. LABORATORY CONSIDERATIONS FOR PROLONGED FUO EVALUATION[a]

Routine

Hct	Uric acid	Direct and indirect bilirubin
WBC	Skin tests: PPD, Candida,	Immunoelectrophoresis
Differential	Trichophyton	
Smear	Chest x-ray	Blood cultures (3–6):
Urine analysis	Sigmoidoscopy	Aerobic and anaerobic
Stool culture and parasites	Sed. rate	Urine culture
Sugar, BUN, HCO_3	VDRL	Sonogram of abdomen + pelvis
Na, K, Cl, Ca	SGOT, Alkaline phosphatase	

If Still No Answer:

LP with appropriate work-up
Bone marrow: biopsy and cultures
Serologies
Liver biopsy
CAT scan/MRI

For More Specific Investigation:

Search for abscess	Search for TB	Search for endocarditis
Sinus x-rays	Gastric aspirates, sputums, urine for TB	Discuss special blood cultures with laboratory
KUB	Liver biopsy with smears and cultures	Echocardiography
		Candida, Aspergillus serology
IVP	Check psoas margins (KUB)	Q fever serology
Gallbladder	IVP	
Barium enema	GI x-rays ↓ Laparoscopy	
Upper GI with small bowel		
Gallium scan	Open liver biopsy ↓ ?Therapeutic trial	
Celiac, renal arteriography		

(continued)

TABLE 1.2. *(continued)*

If Collagen Disease Is Suspected:

Antinuclear and specific antibodies	Biopsy suspicious skin lesions, tender muscles	Renal biopsy
		Sinus x-ray
		↓
Rheumatoid factor	Biopsy of temporal artery	?Therapeutic trial aspirin or steroids
		or
Serum complement	Renal arteriography	Observation

If Occult Tumor Is Suspected:

Apical lordotics	Bone scan and x-rays	Cytology on any obtainable body fluids: peritoneal, pleural
Barium enema	Ultrasonography	
UGI and small bowel follow-through	CAT scan (whole body/MRI)	a-fetoprotein, PSA, 5-HIAA etc.
		↓
Liver Biopsy	Celiac and renal arteriography	Biopsy any affected areas (nodes, liver, skin lesions, lesions, etc.)
Bone marrow biopsy	Echocardiography	
		↓
IVP		Laparotomy or observation

Miscellaneous

Lung scan

Laparoscopy

Other diagnosis made by history or x-rays or biopsies done for other conditions.

(continued)

TABLE 1.2. (continued)

If Epidemiologic or Clinical Clues Are Suggestive, Run Following Serologies		
Monospot, EBV	Rickettsial	Coccidioidomycosis
Toxoplasma	Q fever	Antistreptolysin "O"
CMV	Psittacosis	Cold agglutinins
HBV, HCV	Ameba	Mycoplasma
Brucella	Histoplasma	Trichina
Tularemia		Other viral or parasitic diseases

[a] All these studies are not necessary in each patient but should be considered on the basis of clinical suspicion and data from less invasive procedures.

2

ACUTE PNEUMONITIS

Many different microorganisms can infect the lung and produce pneumonia. Patients with pneumonia usually present with fever, cough, and an infiltrate on chest x-ray. In addition, there may be leukocytosis or leukopenia, chest pain, and varying degrees of respiratory insufficiency. Once pneumonia is suspected, the specific etiologic diagnosis is mandatory, since the choice of treatment is dependent on this information. Although many microbes are capable of producing a pulmonary infiltrate, most cases of pneumonia are caused by one of three or four pulmonary pathogens. A careful history will usually suggest which patient is likely to be infected with one of the less common causes of pneumonia. This discussion will first explore the more common causes of pneumonia and then briefly outline some of the rare etiologies (Table 2.1).

COMMON CAUSES OF PNEUMONIA

In an otherwise healthy patient, the common causes of pneumonia can be predicted in part by the patient's age. As a rule, pneumonia in the healthy child and young adult is caused by mycoplasma or viruses, with bacterial infection more commonly seen in the newborn, the older patient, and those with underlying disease or exposure to a specific pathogen.

TABLE 2.1. ACUTE PNEUMONITIS

A. Common causes of pneumonia[a]
 1. Mycoplasma
 2. Viruses
 3. Bacteria
    a. Pneumococcus
    b. Aspiration pneumonia (mixed)
    c. Gram-negative bacilli
    d. *S. aureus*
    e. *H. influenzae*
    f. *Moraxella*
 4. Tuberculosis
 5. *Chlamydia pneumoniae*

B. Less common causes of pneumonia[b]
 1. Legionnaire's disease
 2. Actinomycosis
 3. Tularemia
 4. Plague
 5. Salmonellosis
 6. Brucellosis
 7. Melioidosis
 8. Q fever
 9. Psittacosis
 10. *Chlamydia trachomatis* (infants)
 11. Fungal infections
    a. Blastomycosis
    b. Coccidioidomycosis
    c. Histoplasmosis
 12. Parasitic infections
    a. *E. histolytica*
    b. Nematodes
    c. Malaria

C. Additional causes of pneumonia in the compromised host[c]
 1. Nocardia
 2. Viruses
    a. CMV
    b. Varicella-zoster
    c. Herpes hominis

TABLE 2.1. *(continued)*

3. Fungi
    a. Candida
    b. Aspergillus
    c. Cryptococcus
    d. Phycomycetes
4. Parasites
    a. Pneumocystis
    b. Toxoplasma
    c. Strongyloides

a Other pulmonary syndromes that must be considered in the differential diagnosis of pulmonary infiltrate in the noncompromised host are (1) pulmonary embolism and (2) pulmonary infiltrates with eosinophilia (PIE syndrome).
b The noncompromised host who has had either certain epidemiologic exposure or who is not responding appropriately to therapy for one of the more common causes of pulmonary infection. At times, specific clinical features in certain of these diseases will suggest the diagnosis.
c Remember, any infection that infects a noncompromised host can also infect this group of patients.

Pneumonia in the newborn is nearly always bacterial in origin. From 2 months to 5 years of age, viruses [respiratory syncytial virus (RSV) and parainfluenza] cause most pneumonia, although in early infancy (1 to 4 months) *Chlamydia trachomatis* is also an important pathogen. Bacteria, especially *H. influenzae*, pneumococci and staphylococci, are less common in this age group but tend to cause severe disease. Then, from age 5 to 30, *Mycoplasma pneumoniae* is the predominant lower respiratory tract pathogen. After age 30, pneumococcal pneumonia again predominates, but Gram-negative rod and staphylococcal pneumonia are also important, as are Legionella and *Chlamydia pneumoniae*.

Mycoplasmal Pneumonia

In the otherwise healthy older child or young adult, the most frequent cause of pneumonia is *M. pneumoniae*. Patients with mycoplasmal pneumonia have a hacking, nonproductive cough and a normal or slightly elevated leukocyte count. Although the physical examination of the chest is usually normal or only mildly abnormal, the chest x-ray may show marked involvement. Early changes on x-ray include a peribronchial interstitial pattern, which may progress to a soft, patchy, lobar consolidation. The latter is localized primarily to the lower lobes, and cavitation is not seen. Pleural involvement usually produces no clinical symptoms, although small pleural effusions may sometimes occur. Mycoplasma infection may cause extra-pulmonic symptoms, such as hepatitis, meningoencephalitis, rash and hemolytic anemia, all potential clues to a mycoplasmal etiology of pneumonitis. It is apparent that although there may be clues to the diagnosis of mycoplasmal pneumonia, nothing about the clinical picture is pathognomonic. When the presentation is fever and a localized infiltrate, mycoplasmal pneumonia can be clinically indistinguishable from viral or other bacterial pneumonias. The diagnosis is usually made serologically.

Mycoplasma is representative of the so-called atypical pneumonias, a clinical entity involving fever, nonproductive cough, constitutional complaints such as myalgias and arthralgias, and a chest x-ray that sometimes shows diffuse interstitial infiltrates. These atypical pneumonias differ from classic bacterial pneumonia in that the latter usually causes a localized infiltrate, productive cough and less in the way of constitutional symptoms. The major causes of atypical pneumonia are Mycoplasma, viruses, Chlamydia, other nonbacterial pathogens, and, on occasion, Legionnaire's disease.

Bacterial Pneumonia

The common bacterial causes of pneumonia include the pneumococci, mouth anerobes, Gram-negative bacilli, and staphylococci. Patients with alcoholism, chronic obstructive pulmonary disease, congestive heart failure, and diabetes are particularly susceptible to bacterial pneumonias, as are patients with the less common problems of multiple myeloma, hypogammaglobulinemia, nephrotic syndrome, and splenectomy. Local factors the presence of which should suggest a bacterial pneumonia are chest trauma, aspiration, bronchiectasis, areas of cystic disease of the lung, and obstructing lesions such as tumors and foreign bodies.

Pneumococcal Pneumonia

The pneumococcus is the most common cause of bacterial pneumonia, especially in nonhospitalized patients. Pneumococcal pneumonia occurs frequently in the setting of a prior viral upper respiratory infection. Typically, there is an explosive onset of a rigor (rigors are rare in nonbacterial pneumonia), cough, pleuritic pain, rusty or purulent sputum, sustained fever, and a consolidation of one or more lobes. Leukocytosis with a marked shift to the left is commonly observed in pneumococcal pneumonia, although a normal leukocyte count is present at times. In severe infection, especially in alcoholic patients, leukopenia occurs and is associated with a grave prognosis. Mortality is low if appropriate therapy is given, and the histologic resolution of the lung is complete. Sterile pleural effusions are common, but empyema is rare with early diagnosis and adequate therapy. Older textbooks stress the observation that pneumococcal pneumonia is frequently introduced by a single rigor, but many clinicians today see this presentation only rarely.

Sometimes the most prominent symptom on presentation is chest pain. Aside from myocardial ischemia and esophageal pain, less common causes of an acutely ill patient with chest pain include pulmonary embolism, herpes zoster, pericarditis, pleurodynia, pleurisy, dissecting aneurysm and sterno-clavicular arthritis.

Staphylococcal and Gram-negative Rod Pneumonia

Staphylococci and Gram-negative rods usually produce a more severe pneumonia, with pleural effusion and empyema occurring more commonly than in pneumococcal infection. The necrotization seen with these more destructive bacterial pneumonias produces an x-ray appearance of infiltrates with areas of abscess formation. However, cavities are also seen with tuberculosis and in mixed anaerobe infections. Pneumococci only rarely produce abscesses, but in patients with severe chronic obstructive pulmonary disease, pneumococcal pneumonia may appear cavitary because of the pre-existing underlying structural disease of the lung.

Staphylococcal Pneumonia

Except during influenza epidemics, when its incidence rises about threefold, staphylococcal pneumonia is uncommon and occurs in less than 5 percent of adult patients admitted to hospitals with bacterial pneumonia. Both the acute bronchopulmonary involvement by the influenza virus and the ravages of chronic obstructive pulmonary disease predispose to pneumonic invasion by staphylococci. Others at risk for staphylococcal pneumonia include (a) children under two years of age, in whom this organism accounts for about one-third of pneumonia deaths, (b) debilitated adults, and (c) patients who develop a metastatic form of staphylococcal pneumonia secondary to bacteremia, usually arising from a focus in the skin, or from an indwelling IV catheter. Metastatic staphylococcal pneumonia also occurs in the IV drug abuser.

Clues suggesting staphylococcal pneumonia include rapidly progressing infiltrates, empyema with early loculation, pneumatoceles, cavitation, spontaneous pneumothorax and cavitary pulmonary emboli.

Gram-negative Bacilli

A variety of these form another relatively common group of etiologic agents producing bacterial pneumonias. Although some investigators have attempted to identify a particular pattern on the chest x-ray for each of the various types of Gram-negative bacilli, we have not found this approach very helpful.

The most common Gram-negative pulmonary pathogen is *Klebsiella spp.*, but *E. coli*, *Pseudomonas spp.*, and *Proteus spp.* may also cause pneumonia. Rarely is a healthy individual affected by these bacteria; most cases appear in those with chronic pulmonary disease, alcoholism, diabetes, or heart disease. In hospitalized patients, respiratory infections are frequently caused by Gram-negative aerobic organisms, especially when mechanical ventilation or tracheostomy has been utilized. Changes in the normal flora by prior antibiotic therapy may also predispose to infection with these organisms. Furthermore, even if none of the above risk factors is present, a seriously ill hospitalized patient has an increased likelihood of being colonized with Gram-negative rods in the oropharynx. Since most pneumonia results from aspiration, it is apparent why Gram-negative pneumonias occur in this setting.

Klebsiella Pneumonia

Certain clinical findings are more characteristic of one Gram-negative pathogen than another. For example, Klebsiella infection should be considered especially in the alcoholic and the malnourished. Leukopenia is not uncommon. The voluminous thick gelatinous fluid produced by Klebsiella may cause a dense infiltrate with lobar enlargement, especially in the upper lobe. A bulging fissure may be present on chest x-ray. At times extensive destruction results in atelectasis of a lobe and the fissure may be bowed inward. This destructive tendency explains the frequent complications related to *K. pneumoniae*, i.e., abscess, pleural effusion, empyema and residual fibrosis. Despite the above clinical clues, Klebsiella pneumonia is usually impossible to differentiate from pneumococcal pneumonia except by Gram stain and culture of sputum, tracheal aspirate, or pleural fluid. Klebsiella pneumonia may sometimes be chronic, simulating tuberculosis or a nonspecific aspiration lung abscess.

Pseudomonas Pneumonia

Pseudomonas pneumonia is particularly a problem in patients with cystic fibrosis, leukemia, or severe leukopenia and in hospitalized patients requiring antibiotics and intensive pulmonary care. Histologically, *P. aeruginosa* is more likely to produce vasculitis with pulmonary vessel thrombosis than are other Gram-negative organisms.

Moraxella catarrhalis, formerly known as *Neisseria catarrhalis*, and then as *Branhamella catarrhalis*, is a Gram-negative diplococcus that has emerged as an important cause of pneumonia in older patients with chronic lung disease.

Anaerobic Pneumonia

There is increasing evidence that a variety of anaerobic bacteria, including anaerobic streptococci and various anaerobic Gram-negative rods, are responsible for a large percentage of bacterial pneumonias. The majority of these lower respiratory infections result from aspiration of normal mouth flora (which consists predominantly of anaerobic bacteria), especially in alcoholic patients or those with other reasons for frequent lapses in consciousness. Patients with bronchogenic carcinoma also are at high risk for anaerobic pneumonia. Anaerobic pneumonia is suggested in these patients, especially if dental hygiene is poor, if the sputum is particularly malodorous, and if the Gram stain of the sputum demonstrates many PMLs and a mixture of Gram-positive and pleomorphic Gram-negative rods resembling mouth flora. In fact, routine aerobic cultures of such material are generally reported as "normal flora." These pneumonias may be fulminant or indolent but necrotization, abscess formation, and empyema are frequently present.

Anaerobic pneumonia may sometimes follow bacteremia, most often related to abdominal surgery, gynecologic infection, or to disruption of the gastrointestinal tract, as from carcinoma (when carcinoma is the underlying disorder, certain organisms such as *Clostridium septicum* provide an etiologic clue). In such situations the pneumonia may present with multiple embolic pulmonary lesions which may cavitate.

Haemophilus Pneumonia

Haemophilus influenzae, although a Gram-negative aerobic rod, should be considered apart from the Gram-negative enteric bacilli or the pseudomonads. The true incidence of pneumonia caused by *H. influenzae* is unknown. The organism may be found as a colonizer in the normal pharyngeal flora of many individuals, but is most frequently observed in young children and in the pharynx or sputum of adults with chronic obstructive pulmonary disease (COPD). These latter two groups of patients are those most likely to develop pneumonia due to *H. influenzae*. The sputum smear shows a predominance of small pleomorphic coccobacillary Gram-negative organisms associated with PMLs. The pneumonia produced by this organism is not distinctive on clinical grounds.

Legionnaire's Disease

Legionnaire's disease produces severe illness and the mortality rate may be as high as 10 to 15 percent in some outbreaks. The patient presents with a history of headache, malaise, and myalgia of brief duration followed by onset of high fever, chills, nonproductive cough, and frequently, gastrointestinal symptoms. Exposure to an excavation site, water (cooling towers, etc.) is common, and in some hospitals Legionella is an important nosocomial pathogen. Except for rales, the physical examination is usually normal. Chest x-rays show patchy infiltrates that progress to widespread consolidations. The disease has been observed to occur in both sporadic and epidemic forms, and most cases occur in adults who smoke. Although the organism is Gram-negative, special stains are usually required for its demonstration, and a fluorescent antibody stain has been found useful. Serologic methods for diagnosis are available and Legionella may be cultured on special media.

Tuberculosis

Mycobacterium tuberculosis remains an important treatable cause of pneumonia. The classic tuberculous lesion occurs in the upper lobe and progresses to cavity formation and scarring. The course is usually indolent and not confused with acute bacterial pneumonia. However, it must be appreciated that there are some acute forms of tuberculosis as well. *M. tuberculosis* can cause an acute pneumonitis, indistinguishable from the pyogenic etiologies already discussed, so that tuberculosis should be considered as a possibility in virtually any pulmonary infiltrative disease. If a patient with a suspected acute bacterial pneumonia fails to respond to antibiotics, the possibility of tuberculosis must be entertained. Other presentations of tuberculosis include the sudden onset of pleural effusion or of infiltrate with ipsilateral hilar adenopathy.

Chlamydia pneumoniae

This organism, also referred to as the TWAR agent, is a common pathogen. Most infections are asymptomatic, but when symptoms occur, children and young adults develop pharyngitis, hoarseness and sinusitis with occasional pneumonia, and adults tend to develop pneumonias. In fact, 10% of pneumonias in patients over 30 may be due to *C. pneumoniae*. Infection with *Chlamydia pneumoniae* often causes persistent symptoms, such as cough and malaise; these may last for weeks or months even with appropriate antibiotic therapy. There may be an association between *Chlamydia pneumoniae* infection and the subsequent onset of asthma.

Laboratory Diagnosis of Bacterial Pneumonia

Since neither clinical nor radiologic findings can specifically diagnose the etiology of most pneumonias, other laboratory methods represent more important tools to the clinician. The most helpful tests available are blood cultures, sputum Gram stains, and cultures of sputum and pleural fluid. In fact, a positive blood or pleural fluid culture is the most definitive method of identifying the causative agent unless culture of the lung tissue itself can be performed. Unfortunately, blood cultures are positive in only about one-fourth of the cases of pneumonia, except in those infections of the lung that are metastatic and secondary to bacteremia from another source.

The sputum smear is invaluable if it shows many inflammatory cells (usually polymorphs) and a uniformity of flora, i.e., all Gram-positive cocci or Gram-negative rods. The organisms should be near or inside the polymorphs to be significant.

Culture of the sputum alone is less helpful than the Gram stain for several reasons. Anaerobic cocci and rods, pneumococci, staphylococci, streptococci, Haemophilus and Branhamella may all be part of the normal flora cultured from the nasopharynx. Furthermore, Gram-negative rods are not infrequently found in the upper airway of severely ill, hospitalized patients. Thus, the mere demonstration of an organism in a sputum culture without a concomitant Gram stain showing evidence of PMLs, pulmonary macrophages, and a predominant type of bacterial flora provides little help to the clinician. In addition, failure to culture pneumococci from sputum of patients with pneumococcal pneumonia (proven by positive blood culture) occurs frequently enough to indicate the hazard of interpreting sputum cultures without the results of Gram stains.

There are several problems encountered in Gram stains of sputums. First, one must be sure one is looking at sputum and not primarily at saliva. The best proof that the specimen is sputum is the presence of the alveolar macrophage. Areas with large numbers of epithelial cells should not be studied since they represent material derived from the upper airway. Second, the quality of the stain can be checked by observation of the color of the nucleus of the PML, which should be light pink rather than blue. To check for proper decolorization, a control made with known Gram-negative and Gram-positive organisms may be run. A sample of one's own teeth tartar, which should contain both Gram-positive and Gram-negative bacteria, makes an excellent control when performing a Gram stain. Finally, areas in which numerous PMLs are present should be selected for careful examination for bacteria. In active infection, PMLs containing ingested bacteria are sometimes seen. The presence of large numbers of intraleukocytic Gram-positive cocci suggest that the organisms are more likely staphylococci than pneumococci, since (a) these latter, usually heavily-encapsulated bacteria, are phagocytized with difficulty in early infection (prior to the development of specific antibody) and (b) once ingested, pneumococci are readily killed.

The finding of numerous PMLs and mixed flora on the Gram stain with many pleomorphic Gram-negative rods that fail to grow aerobically is a most helpful clue in the diagnosis of anaerobic pneumonia. The presence of many inflammatory cells with a relative paucity of bacteria suggests either a nonbacterial process or infection due to a bacterium not seen on Gram stain. Mycoplasma and Legionnaire's disease should be strongly considered in this situation, although other important etiologies include tuberculosis, viral pneumonia, Q fever, psittacosis, and chlamydia.

Molecular biologic techniques such as DNA probes and polymerase chain reaction (PCR) are being applied to sputum for the diagnosis of pneumonia. A growing variety of pathogens including fungi, mycobacteria, bacteria and viruses is being subjected to these recently-developed tests; the usefulness of these new modalities will depend on their commercial availability to the general clinician, and their cost.

Although microscopic examination of the expectorated sputum is a very helpful noninvasive technique that often suggests the etiologic agent, it may be necessary to employ other diagnostic procedures. A transtracheal aspirate is occasionally useful in bypassing nasopharyngeal contamination and in obtaining sputum from a patient unable to expectorate. Bronchoscopy and nasopharyngeal suction reach below the normally sterile carina and are less invasive than transtracheal aspiration, although pharyngeal contamination is inevitable with these techniques.

Finally, some points about the treatment of pneumonia should be stressed. In general, the antimicrobial treatment of pneumonia is based on the etiology suggested by appropriate Gram stains. At times, treatment must be instituted without a good sputum smear or other laboratory aids. In these situations, treatment should be planned with the likely etiologies in mind. For example, in an otherwise healthy college student with a nonproductive cough, fever, and a localized infiltrate, who does not appear too ill, one would suspect primarily a mycoplasmal pneumonia. On occasion, pneumococci or viruses are the culprits. Erythromycin could be used to treat both mycoplasma and pneumococci in this setting. On the other hand, if a patient is seriously ill, with multiple infiltrates, hypoxia, and high fever, it is imperative to obtain sputum for a Gram stain. But if the results are still inconclusive, initial antibiotic coverage should include agents effective against staphylococci and Gram-negative bacilli, in addition to pneumococci, anaerobes and possibly Legionnella. Additional etiologic considerations have to include the patient's age, immune status, and exposure to possible specific pathogens.

OTHER CAUSES OF PNEUMONIA

Pneumonias are caused by other agents, including a variety of viruses, fungi, and parasites. Other than the viruses, these etiologies are all much less frequent than the infections already discussed. But they merit consideration when certain clinical and epidemiologic factors exist or when pneumonia, thought to be secondary to one of the common bacterial etiologies, fails to respond to appropriate therapy. In young infants, *Chlamydia trachomatis* is an important cause of pneumonia which at times is associated with very little or no fever.

Viral Pneumonia

Viral pneumonias may be caused by influenza, parainfluenza, adenovirus (especially in epidemics in a close population, e.g., the military), RSV, and, less frequently, by varicella, rubeola, and the herpes viruses. In general, constitutional symptoms predominate, with fever, headache, dry cough, malaise, and myalgias. The leukocyte count is usually normal or slightly low, but neutrophilia with significant polymorphonuclear leukocytosis is sometimes present. In severe cases, dyspnea and marked hypoxia may occur. Although cough and purulent sputum are usually suggestive of bacterial infection, these symptoms are occasionally seen with severe viral pneumonia such as influenza. The symptoms of viral pneumonia may be dramatic and the x-ray changes extensive despite minimal findings on physical examination of the chest. The most common x-ray appearance is a patchy lower-lobe segmental consolidation, limited to one lobe, frequently similar to the findings observed in most bacterial pneumonia. Minimal atelectasis may be present. Other x-ray patterns are more suggestive of viral infection, but are seen less commonly; they include an interstitial pattern radiating from the hilar areas or a diffuse symmetric pattern throughout both lungs that is either interstitial or nodular. Thus the pattern may be indistinguishable from pulmonary edema or interstitial fibrosis. Pleural involvement from the aforementioned viruses is rare, explaining the infrequency of pleuritic pain and pleural effusion with viral pneumonia. Cavitation does not occur.

A few of the individual viral pneumonias produce findings that are characteristic but by no means pathognomonic. The herpes viruses (varicella-zoster, herpes simplex type 1, and CMV) often cause a diffusely symmetric pattern of consolidation. Varicella is frequently diffusely nodular and may leave a residuum of multiple 1 to 3 mm calcifications. Influenza can produce any form of infiltration on x-ray. In adenovirus, a hazy segmental consolidation is the most common x-ray pattern seen, just as it is in influenza pneumonia. In newborns and infants, RSV may cause a severe form of pneumonia and may be epidemic in nurseries.

The diffuse patchy infiltrate described in classic viral pneumonias may also be seen in (a) nonviral pneumonias, (b) septicemia, (c) acute aspiration, and (d) pulmonary edema of diverse etiologies.

Clinical suspicion of viral pneumonia may be raised by a pneumonitis that fails to respond to antibiotics and by normal or slightly low white blood cell (WBC) counts. Also, appropriate sputum stains may demonstrate inclusions within inflammatory cells or the presence of multinucleated giant cells, which suggests the presence of certain viral pneumonias. Definitive diagnosis is based on viral cultures and appropriate serologies.

Epidemiologic Clues to Etiology

Other etiologic agents that are infrequently encountered include Rickettsia, Leptospira, Toxoplasma, some parasites, fungi, and the organisms responsible for tularemia, plague, typhoid fever, and brucellosis. These occur primarily in characteristic epidemiologic settings, and careful questioning of the patient concerning living habits, travel, diet, and pets may help significantly in diagnosis. For example, Q fever should be suspected in slaughterhouse workers who have been exposed to infected animals. The infiltrates are usually patchy and segmental, and frequently hepatitis and myalgias are seen. Unlike other rickettsial diseases, rash is absent in Q fever. Splenomegaly, bradycardia, and a rash resembling "rose spots" should suggest psittacosis in a patient with exposure to birds. Exposure to ticks, biting flies, or to animals like muskrats and rabbits may help point to the diagnosis of tularemic pneumonia. These patients are extremely ill, and pleural involvement is pronounced. Infection with *Yersinia pestis*, the cause of plague, may involve the lungs and produce a severe pneumonia that is extremely contagious if the organism is found in the sputum. Since it is spread by the rat flea, exposure to rats and other rodents in an area of high endemicity is important. In the United States, plague is rare, but the disease is seen every year in the Southwest, where it is endemic in rodents.

Pneumonia in the Compromised Host

Another group of patients who may develop pneumonias of unusual etiology are those who have a serious disturbance in their host-defense mechanism, e.g., immunosuppression resulting from a disease such as AIDS (see Chapter 13) or Hodgkin's disease, or from medications such as cancer chemotherapy. In this setting, less common organisms need special consideration. The protozoan *Pneumocystis carinii* may cause a pneumonitis associated with fever, cough, and progressive dyspnea and tachypnea. Physical findings are often minimal. The chest x-ray may show a wide spectrum of findings, but most characteristic is a bilateral diffuse or patchy infiltration. If untreated, death from hypoxia is likely. Other opportunistic organisms that need to be considered in these patients include fungi (especially Aspergillus, Candida, Phycomycetes, and Cryptococcus), bacteria (such as Nocardia and Legionella), and certain viruses (particularly herpes simplex type 1 and CMV).

The chest x-ray findings produced by these unusual organisms are once again not highly specific, and diagnosis depends on visualization or culture of the pathogen. Though expectorated sputums should be examined, they are not very helpful in many instances. Thus, immunosuppressed patients with pneumonia usually require more invasive diagnostic techniques than their immunologically competent counterparts. Bronchoscopy with brush biopsy or lung biopsy with appropriate smears, stains, and cultures are very helpful tools. Since most of these infections can be treated with specific antimicrobial drugs, rapid etiologic diagnosis is imperative. Infections with these organisms are discussed in greater detail in Chapter 12, Infection in the Compromised Host.

Finally, noninfectious causes of pulmonary infiltrate may resemble pneumonia, especially when accompanied by fever. These are listed in Table 2.2.

TABLE 2.2. NONINFECTIOUS CAUSES OF PULMONARY INFILTRATE

A. Common Causes
   1. Pulmonary embolus
   2. Aspiration
   3. Tumor-primary or metastatic
   4. Congestive heart failure

B. Less Common Causes
   1. Sarcoid
   2. Pneumoconiosis
   3. Extrinsic allergic alveolitis
   4. Alveolar proteinosis
   5. Desquamative interstitial pneumonitis
   6. Irradiation injury
   7. Vasculitis
   8. Sickle cell pneumopathy
   9. Therapeutic agents (e.g., bleomycin or nitrofurantoin)
   10. Oxygen toxicity or shock lung

TABLE 2.3.—DIAGNOSTIC CHART: ACUTE PNEUMONITIS—SELECTED ETIOLOGIES

Acute Pneumonitis

Organism	Etiology, Epidemiology, and/or Pathogenesis	Clinical Signs	Diagnosis	Initial Treatment
A. Common Causes				
1. *M. pneumoniae*	Respiratory spread. Usually introduced into the family by small children.	Nonproductive cough. May show lobar (usually lower lobe) or diffuse involvement. Pulse-temperature dissociation sometimes present. Pleurisy uncommon. WBC usually normal or only minimally increased.	Special pharyngeal or sputum cultures required for mycoplasma isolation. Serology (mycoplasma and cold agglutinins). PCR may ultimately prove helpful.	Erythromycin (doxycycline)
2. Viruses	Common viral infections in the nonimmunosuppressed individual: adenovirus, influenza, parainfluenza, RSV, varicella.	Constitutional signs may predominate, chest x-ray may show diffuse interstitial pattern, but usually shows the disease confined to one lower lobe. In severe cases, marked hypoxia may occur.	Viral cultures from throat. Acute and convalescent serum.	Influenza—amantidine, rimantidine Varicella—acyclovir Herpes hominis—acyclovir CMV—ganciclovir

ACUTE PNEUMONITIS

3. *Streptococcus pneumoniae*	Aspiration.	Most common cause of bacterial pneumonia in the adult. Explosive onset. May be lobar or bronchopneumonia. Pleurisy common. Productive cough. Herpes labialis may be seen. Rapid response to penicillin.	Blood culture. Smear and cultures of sputum, pleural fluid.	Penicillin G (Erythromycin or cephalosporin). Penicillin-resistant strains should be treated with cefotaxime for moderate resistance and vancomycin for high-grade resistance.
4. *Staphylococcus aureus*	May result from aspiration or from hematogenous spread. At high risk are infants, IV drug abusers, patients with influenza, or patients with staphylococcal tricuspid endocarditis.	Rapidly progressing infiltrates. Empyema common with early loculation. Pneumatoceles. Cavitation. Spontaneous pneumothorax. Multiple lobe involvement. Anemia.	Blood culture. Smear and culture of pleural fluid (if present). Sputum smear (showing Gram-positive cocci within PMNs) and culture.	Vancomycin Initially. If methicillin-susceptible and patient not allergic to penicillin, nafcillin would then be treatment of choice.
5. *H. influenzae*	Seen especially in infants and in patients with COPD.	Not distinctive	Blood culture. Smear and culture of sputum. Smear and culture of pleural fluid if present.	2nd or 3rd generation cephalosporin should be used unless isolate shown to be ampicillin-sensitive.

(continued)

TABLE 2.3. *(continued)* **DIAGNOSTIC CHART: ACUTE PNEUMONITIS**

Acute Pneumonitis

Organism	Etiology, Epidemiology, and/or Pathogenesis	Clinical Signs	Diagnosis	Initial Treatment
6. Gram-negative bacilli	Pneumonia may result from either aspiration of gram-negative rods that have colonized the throat or from bacteremia secondary to infection at a distant site such as the urinary tract. Rarely seen in healthy ambulatory adults. Usually either nosocomial or occurring in patients with alcoholism, diabetes, chronic lung disease, or other problems of host defense.	May resemble pneumococcal pneumonia completely. Multiple lobes frequently involved. Unlike pneumococcal pneumonia, cavity formation and empyema commonly occur.	Blood culture. Smear and culture of sputum. Smear and culture of pleural fluid if present.	Aminoglycoside plus piperacillin or aminoglycoside plus ceftazidime until cultures available.
a. *K. pneumonia*	Particularly seen in alcoholics.	Upper lobe commonly involved; both acute and chronic forms are seen. Bulging fissure may be present on x-ray.	Blood culture. Smear and cultures of sputum. Smear and culture of pleural fluid if present.	3rd generation cephalosporin.
b. *P. aeruginosa*	Aspiration of colonizing organisms resulting in	Abscess formation very common. Some	Blood culture. Smear and culture of sputum.	Tobramycin and piperacillin or

ACUTE PNEUMONITIS

	pneumonia. Almost always nosocomial, especially in patients with endotracheal tubes. Also seen in patients with cystic fibrosis, hematologic tumors, and/or with granulocytopenia.	investigators state that relative bradycardia and reversal of diurnal temperatures curve is common.	Smear and culture of pleural fluid if present.	gentamicin and piperacillin or amikacin and piperacillin.
7. Anaerobic pneumonia a. Aspiration	Aspiration.	Aspiration may be followed by an acute pneumonia or a chronic non-specific abscess. Sputum smells foul and patients report bad taste in mouth. X-ray may show necrotizing pneumonia, pulmonary edema pattern or abscess formation. On occasion, aspiration of sterile material (e.g., vomitus) may simulate bacterial infection with cough dyspnea, infiltrate and fever.	Blood cultures. Sputum smear and aerobic culture show no predominant pathogens, but reflect "mouth flora," with fusobacteria, gram-positive cocci, gram-negative pleomorphic rods, and spirochetes. Although not usually necessary, if a transtracheal aspirate is done, it should be cultured both aerobically and anaerobically. Smear d culture pleural fluid if present (both aerobically and anaerobically).	Clindamycin or ampicillin—sulbactam. Also useful: metronidazole, piperacillin— Tazobactam, and Ticarcillin—clavulanate

(continued)

TABLE 2.3. (continued) DIAGNOSTIC CHART: ACUTE PNEUMONITIS

Acute Pneumonitis

Organism	Etiology, Epidemiology, and/or Pathogenesis	Clinical Signs	Diagnosis	Initial Treatment
b. Metastatic	Bacteremia from pelvic or GI focus seen especially with pelvic infection or with GI cancer or surgery.	Necrotizing with frequent cavitation and empyema formation. Infiltrates are often multiple resembling pulmonary emboli.	Blood cultures. Sputum smear usually shows predominance of pleomorphic Gram-negative rods. Only a transtracheal aspirate should be cultured for anaerobes, not expectorated specimens. Smear and culture of pleural fluid.	As above
c. Lung Abscess	Aspiration of mixed aerobic or anaerobic mouth flora or aspiration of specific aerobic organisms known to have tendency to cause abscesses such as (1) S.	May produce copious sputum if abscess communicates with a bronchus. Hemorrhage not infrequent. If anaerobic, may be very foul smelling.	Blood culture helpful in metastatic infection. Sputum smear and aerobic culture show no predominant pathogens, but reflect "mouth flora," with fusobacteria,	Drainage and antimicrobial therapy. Antibiotic therapy as above is indicated if aspiration of mouth anaerobes is suspected on basis of Gram

ACUTE PNEUMONITIS

	aureus or (2) Gram-negative rods. At times related to an underlying carcinoma with abscess or to a septic embolization from a distant focus of infection.		Gram-positive cocci, Gram-negative pleomorphic rods, and spirochetes. Although not usually necessary, if a transtracheal aspirate is done, it should be cultured both aerobically and anaerobically. Smear and culture pleural fluid if present (both aerobically and anaerobically).	stain. Otherwise, treat on basis of suspected etiologic agent as noted on Gram stain.
8. *M. tuberculosis* a. Primary	Airborne droplets usually produce asymptomatic infection.	If infection is limited, a peripheral lung infiltrate with unilateral hilar adenopathy may appear that clears, leaving only a Ghon complex. Minimal to no symptoms or signs. Seen especially in young children.	If limited, skin test (PPD) conversion occurs by 6 weeks and may be all that is noted.	Isoniazid prophylaxis given for primary infection manifested only by skin-test conversion (i.e., no progressive disease). For prophylaxis of multidrug resistant TB (MDR-TB): PZA + ofloxacin. For prophylaxis of INH-resistant organisms: RIF + ETH.

(continued)

TABLE 2.3. (continued) DIAGNOSTIC CHART: ACUTE PNEUMONITIS

Acute Pneumonitis

Organism	Etiology, Epidemiology, and/or Pathogenesis	Clinical Signs	Diagnosis	Initial Treatment
b. Progressive primary or reinfection (reactivation of dormant focus)	1. May get subacute or chronic infiltrate with or without cavity formation and scarring, usually in the apical region. 2. May get bronchogenic spread and widespread involvement. 3. May get hematogenous spread with systemic organ involvement or miliary dissemination.	1. Fever, coughing, either productive or nonproductive, hemoptysis, night sweats, and weight loss, progressing subacutely. 2. Bronchogenic spread frequently resembles acute bacterial pneumonia. 3. Miliary spread causes high fever, hypoxia, dyspnea, frequently with little cough. At times there is no evidence of disease on the chest x-ray at time of admission. Meningitis is present in a significant number of patients with miliary TB.	Skin test (PPD). Sputum smear (Gram stain and AFB) and culture. Gastric aspirates. In miliary tuberculosis, marrow and liver biopsy for histology and culture are especially helpful. CSF examination should be performed in all suspected cases of miliary tuberculosis. DNA probes and PCR may prove helpful in Dx of TB.	Isoniazid (INH) + rifampin (RIF) + ethambutol (ETH) + pyrazinamide (PZA). For multidrug-resistant (MDR-TB), treat pending culture results with amikacin, ofloxocin, ETH and PZA and possibly additional drugs.

9. *C. pneumoniae*	Common Cause of atypical pneumonia in older patients and of hoarseness, pharyngitis, sinusitis in young patients.	Sinusitis, pharyngitis, hoarseness, wheezing. May see interstitial infiltration. Symptoms may be persistent.	Clinical findings and serology	Erythromycin, doxycycline
B. Less Common causes of pneumonia				
1. Legionnaire's agent	Soil and contaminated cooling towers have been implicated, as well as institutional and recreational water sources.	Symptoms include fever, chills, nonproductive cough, myalgias, abdominal pain, and gastrointestinal, and CNS complaints. X-ray shows diffuse interstitial infiltrates or multiple areas of consolidation.	Culture sputum, pleural fluid on specialized media; Serology; Direct immunofluorescence antibody performed on sputum, tracheal secretions, pleural fluid, or lung biopsies is of great help. Urinary antigen is detectable for *L. pneumophila* Serotype 1. DNA probes helpful when available.	Erythromycin ± rifampin.

(continued)

TABLE 2.3. (continued) DIAGNOSTIC CHART: ACUTE PNEUMONITIS

Acute Pneumonitis

Organism	Etiology, Epidemiology, and/or Pathogenesis	Clinical Signs	Diagnosis	Initial Treatment
2. *Actinomyces israelii*	Organisms present in normal mouth flora. Pneumonia secondary to aspiration. Associated with poor oral hygiene.	Subacute basilar consolidation. Abscess formation may occur with draining sinuses. Can involve pleura and ribs.	Look for sulfur granules in sputum or chest drainage. (these are sometimes found by washing the exudate through a sterile gauze pad or picking yellow granules from drainage dressings; granule should be crushed and Gram stained.) Branching gram-positive filaments seen on smears that do not grow aerobically; acid-fast stains generally negative. Biopsy with smears and cultures. If cultures obtained, must be either transtracheal or from draining lesion or from involved tissue. Fluorescent antibody may help with specific identification on cultures or smear of pus.	Penicillin G or doxycycline.

ACUTE PNEUMONITIS

3. *Francisella tularensis*	Infection acquired from contact with infected animals, especially rabbits and muskrats, or insect vector such as ticks and deerflies. Pneumonia may occur by inhalation, but more commonly is secondary to bacteremia.	Ulceroglandular is the most common form. Cases with pneumoia are most severe. Multiple patches of bronchopneumonia occur frequently with pleural involvement and granulomata on pleural biopsy. Severe toxicity and respiratory distress present. WBC is usually normal. No response to penicillin or cephalosporin.	Gram stain of sputum shows small Gram-negative coccobacillary organisms. Fluorescent antibody stain is very sensitive, specific, and helpful for rapid diagnosis. Culture sputum and blood on special enriched media. Titers rise late.	Streptomycin (doxycycline)
4. *Yersinia pestis*	Bite of the rat flea, with pneumonia secondary to bacteremia or respiratory acquisition by droplet spread from a patient with pneumonic plague. In US, most cases occur in the Southwest, especially among people in close contact with nature.	Severe toxicity and bubo usually evident. Bloody, frothy sputum present in some pneumonic cases. Epidemiologic clues very helpful in diagnosis.	Gram stain of sputum, blood or pus shows short, plump gram-negative rods. Giemsa (bipolar staining) stains are also helpful. Culture on blood agar. Fluorescent antibody stains on tissue specimens, pus or cultures very helpful. Serology is helpful.	Streptomycin. (sensitivity studies are mandatory. Streptomycin-resistant organisms are common in some areas of the world, and other agents such as tetracycline or chloramphenicol may be alternative.)

(continued)

TABLE 2.3. *(continued)* **DIAGNOSTIC CHART: ACUTE PNEUMONITIS**

Acute Pneumonitis

Organism	Etiology, Epidemiology, and/or Pathogenesis	Clinical Signs	Diagnosis	Initial Treatment
5. Salmonella	Rare cause of pneumonia.	Lobar consolidation.	Culture blood, sputum, stool and urine.	Ceftriaxone (quinolone)
6. Brucella	Part of generalized infection. History of animal contact important.	Nondescript x-ray appearance. WBC usually low, with relative lymphocytosis, but may be elevated in severe pneumonia.	Gram stain shows very small coccobacillary gram-negative rods that require special media to grow and a 2–10% CO_2 environment. Sputum and blood should be cultured and cultures of bone marrow are also helpful. Cultures must be kept at least 30 days. Serology very helpful. Fluorescent antibody specific and helpful for staining of tissues.	Doxycycline + Rifampin

ACUTE PNEUMONITIS

7. *Pseudomonas pseudomallei*	Meliodosis seen in U.S., principally in returnees from Southeast Asia or laboratory workers.	May cause an acute pneumonia or a chronic infiltrate that resembles tuberculosis, with upper lobe density and cavitation.	Gram stain, culture and serology	Doxycycline
8. Q fever agent (*Coxiella burneti*)	Q fever is a disease of livestock. Human infection occurs either from inhalation of dust-laden air near infected animals or from tick vectors. Seen in slaughter-house workers and in people who drink unpasteurized milk.	Generalized symptoms include myalgias, headaches, chills, and fever. Cough not productive. *No rash* (unlike other Rickettsia). X-ray variable, usually patchy and segmental. Accompanying hepatitis is common.	Serology	Doxycycline
9. Psittacosis (*Chlamydia psittaci*)	Psittacosis is an infection of birds, transmitted by inhalation of dust-containing feces of infected birds. Seen in many varieties of birds, especially turkeys, parrots, and parakeets.	Fever, cough, severe headache, myalgias, relative bradycardia. "Rose spots," splenomegaly, and epistaxis common. Thrombophlebitis may occur during convalescence. X-ray shows patchy areas of consolidation, though can be diffuse or even miliary.	Serology. Inclusion bodies in mononuclear cells in alveolar exudate, lungs, and spleen. Lugol iodine solution may help stain intracellular inclusions. Giemsa and Macchiavello stains helpful. Dangerous to handle infected specimens, but may be cultured in embryonated eggs and mice.	Doxycycline (erythromycin)

(continued)

TABLE 2.3. (continued) DIAGNOSTIC CHART: ACUTE PNEUMONITIS

Acute Pneumonitis

Organism	Etiology, Epidemiology, and/or Pathogenesis	Clinical Signs	Diagnosis	Initial Treatment
10. *Chlamydia trachomatis* (Infection of Infants)	May be acquired at time of delivery.	Cough, widespread pneumonia.	Serology	Erythromycin
11. Fungi	Some fungi (Aspergillus, Candida, Phycomycetes) cause disease primarily in immunocompromised individuals, while others (Cryptococcus) afflict both normal and immunocompromised hosts; still other organisms (Blastomyces, Coccidioides, Histoplasma) affect predominantly normal	See below.	The presence of Histoplasma, Coccidioides, or Blastomyces in the sputum almost always means actual infection and not mere colonization.	

individuals. These last infections should be considered when the patient lives or has lived in an endemic area or has an appropriate epidemiologic association.

a. *Blastomyces dermatitidis* | Inhalation of organisms, probably from contaminated soil. Usually affects normal individuals. | Primary: mild respiratory symptoms with fleeting infiltrates. Can become progressive and chest x-ray may show pneumonia, para-hilar mass, tumor, and/or cavitation. Cutaneous lesions or osseous lesions (especially in the ribs) may be clues, since these are common sites of metastatic infection. | Silver stain of sputum, bronchial washings, or biopsy of lung lesion. Appropriate fungal cultures. Serology. Prostatic secretions and skin or bone biopsies may also be smeared and cultured. DNA probes may prove useful. | Amphotericin B for progressive disease. Possibly useful: itraconazole.

(continued)

TABLE 2.3. *(continued)* DIAGNOSTIC CHART: ACUTE PNEUMONITIS

Acute Pneumonitis

Organism	Etiology, Epidemiology, and/or Pathogenesis	Clinical Signs	Diagnosis	Initial Treatment
b. *Coccidioides immitis*	Inhalation of spores in endemic area of Southwest U.S. Usually affects normal individuals.	Primary: mild respiratory symptoms associated with hilar nodes and unilateral infiltrate. Can see erythema nodosum, erythema multiforme and eosinophilia for 2–3 weeks after fever disappears. Progressive form: resembles tuberculosis. Suspect with progressive consolidation, with fibrosis and thin-walled cavities in the upper lobes. Bone, joint, or meninges are common	Silver stain of sputum, bronchial washings, or biopsy of lung lesion. Appropriate fungal cultures. Serology. In dissemination, biopsy with stains and cultures of involved tissues may be required for diagnosis. DNA probes may prove useful.	Amphotericin B for progressive disease. Possibly useful: itraconazole.

ACUTE PNEUMONITIS

c. *Histoplasma capsulatum*	Inhalation of organisms from soil contaminated with excreta of various birds such as chickens, starlings, and blackbirds, and of bats. Usually affects normal hosts.	Primary: mild respiratory symptoms. X-ray may show localized or scattered multiple, uniform nodular lesions. Can become progressive and resemble tuberculosis and cause marked fibrosis. At times mucous membranes in mouth and throat are involved and show granulomatous lesions and ulcers. May disseminate throughout RE system and other viscera. May show disseminated calcified lesions in chest and spleen.	Silver stain of sputum, bronchial washings, or biopsy of lung lesion. Appropriate fungal cultures, serology. Bone marrow is a good source for smear and culture, as this organism commonly is found in this tissue. In suspected disseminated disease, peripheral blood, bone marrow, or other involved tissues should be rapidly smeared and cultured. DNA probes may prove useful.	Amphotericin B for progressive disease. Possibly useful: Itraconazole.

(continued)

TABLE 2.3. *(continued)* **DIAGNOSTIC CHART: ACUTE PNEUMONITIS**

Acute Pneumonitis

Organism	Etiology, Epidemiology, and/or Pathogenesis	Clinical Signs	Diagnosis	Initial Treatment
12. Parasites				
a. *Entamoeba histolytica*	Complication of amebic abscess of the liver.	RLL infiltrates; effusion or abscess may occur.	Serology positive in 90% of patients. Sputum may be chocolate-colored with bitter taste. Pleural fluid may show thick exudate with negative bacterial cultures. Amebae should be looked for, though they are rarely seen. Liver involvement is almost always present, with abnormal alkaline phosphatase and a positive liver scan.	Metronidazole
b. Nematodes (*Ascaris*, *Strongyloides*,	During passage through the lungs, may see pulmonary symptoms.	Bronchitis, cough, hemoptysis, pleural effusion, transient	May see larvae in sputum or pleural fluid, but examine stool for	Ancylostoma: mebendazole. Ascaris: piperazine,

ACUTE PNEUMONITIS

ancylostoma, and *Necatur*)		bronchopneumonia, and fever may be present. Eosinophilia, abdominal distress, and diarrhea are commonly noted.	adult worms, eggs, and larvae.	mebendazole. Necatur: mebendazole. Strongyloides: thiabendazole.
c. Malaria (*Plasmodium falciparum*)	Resistant malaria is found in parts of Southeast Asia, Africa, and in South America	Dyspnea, hypoxia, and pulmonary infiltrates present in patient very ill with fever, hemolysis and splenomegaly.	Look for organisms in peripheral blood smear.	Choroquine. If resistance suspected, quinine + Doxycycline (parenteral: IV Quinidine + Cleocin).
C. Causes in the immunocompromised				
1. *Nocardia*	Organism found in soil. Associated with administration of corticosteroids, malignancy, especially lymphoma, and alveolar proteinosis. About 50% of nocardial disease occurs in normal individuals.	On x-ray resembles tuberculosis or bacterial pneumonia. Look for evidence of dissemination to the CNS and bone especially.	Gram stain shows gram-positive branching rods; acidfast stain positive with weak decolorization. Sputum or bronchial washings culture. Biopsy with smears and cultures may be needed if other tests negative.	Sulfonamides (trimethoprim-sulfamethoxazole or minocycline).

(continued)

TABLE 2.3. (continued) DIAGNOSTIC CHART: ACUTE PNEUMONITIS

Acute Pneumonitis

Organism	Etiology, Epidemiology, and/or Pathogenesis	Clinical Signs	Diagnosis	Initial Treatment
2. Fungi				
a. *Candida albicans*	Part of normal pharyngeal and gut flora. Causes pneumonia by aspiration. The most frequent opportunist of all the fungi. Seen with blood dyscrasias, debility, antibiotic and corticosteroid or immunosuppressive treatment, cancer, and surgery.	Resembles other forms of pneumonia. Not responsive to usual antibiotics.	Smear and culture of sputum difficult to interpret. Need material from infected tissue itself, although transtracheal aspirate may be helpful.	Amphotericin B. 5-fluorocytosine may be added if organism is sensitive. Possible alternative: fluconazole.
b. *Aspergillus*	Ubiquitous in nature. May cause severe pulmonary infection as opportunist, e.g., in patients with leukemia or with	Chest x-ray may resemble tumor, bronchopneumonia or abscess.	Culture reliable only if from lung tissue itself. Frequently sputum culture fails to show organisms in patients	Amphotericin B if evidence of progressive infiltrative disease is present.

ACUTE PNEUMONITIS

	immunosuppression. In certain patients may cause allergic manifestations with asthma, wheezing, high IgE titer, + skin test, and sometimes + serology. May also produce a mycetoma in patients with pre-existing cavities.	with pneumonia. Septate hyphae are seen on lung biopsy. Serology. Skin test helpful for diagnosis of bronchopulmonary aspergillosis.	
c. *Cryptococcus neoformans*	Inhalation of organisms found in soil, especially contaminated with pigeon feces. Disease can affect normal individuals, but cryptococci especially produce infection in patients with diabetes, AIDS, lymphoproliferative diseases, or those receiving corticosteroids or cytotoxic agents.	Subacute course common. Pulmonary lesion may resemble "coin lesion," tumor, or pneumonitis. May disseminate, especially to the meninges.	Culture blood, CSF, sputum, and urine. Smear and biopsy specimen (use mucicarmine stain, specific for capsule). Serology. India ink preparations helpful if meninges are involved and are helpful with other specimens.	Amphotericin B and 5-flurocytosine (fluconazole).

(continued)

TABLE 2.3. (continued) DIAGNOSTIC CHART: ACUTE PNEUMONITIS

Acute Pneumonitis

Organism	Etiology, Epidemiology, and/or Pathogenesis	Clinical Signs	Diagnosis	Initial Treatment
d. *Phycomycetes*	Seen especially in leukemia and lymphoma patients	Dense infiltrate with infarction and abscess formation.	Biopsy of lung with appropriate smears and cultures. Wide branching nonseptate hyphae noted with evidence of tissue and vascular invasion.	Amphotericin B. Surgery usually required to remove diseased tissue.
3. *P. carinii*	Seen mostly in patients with AIDS (Chapter 13) but cases also occur in infants or in patients with lymphoreticular malignancy receiving corticosteroids.	Severe dyspnea and hypoxia. Diffuse patchy infiltrates	Stain specimens with silver stain or direct fluorescent stain. Specimens that can be obtained listed from least to most	Trimethoprim-sulfamethoxazole (v. chapter 13).

4. Toxoplasma gondii	May be acquired by ingestion of raw meat. Cats are known to be cyst passers.	Chest x-ray shows a variety of types of infiltrates. Not diagnostic except by serology and lung biopsy. Serology. Lung biopsy with Wright's or Giemsa's stain (best for trophozoites) or PAS stain (for cysts).	Pyrimethamine + sulfadiazine.
5. Viruses	Common in immunosuppressed host: H. hominis, varicella-zoster, CMV.	Diffuse interstitial pneumonia, with dyspnea and marked hypoxia. Biopsy of lung may show viral inclusions with special stains. Cultures and acute and convalescent serum.	H. hominis: Acyclovir V-Z: Acyclovir CMV: Ganciclovir

(continued)

50 DIFFERENTIAL DIAGNOSIS OF INFECTIOUS DISEASES

TABLE 2.3. *(continued)* DIAGNOSTIC CHART: ACUTE PNEUMONITIS

Acute Pneumonitis

Organism	Etiology, Epidemiology, and/or Pathogenesis	Clinical Signs	Diagnosis	Initial Treatment
D. Pulmonary Syndromes Confused with Pneumonia				
1. Pulmonary embolism	Frequently secondary to thrombophlebitis from pelvic, prostatic, or leg veins. Hypercoagulable states, prolonged bed rest, sepsis, and medications such as oral contraceptives are also predisposing factors.	Sudden dyspnea, chest pain, and, at times, hemoptysis. Fever may be present. This entity is frequently confused with infections and should be considered in every patient with suspected pneumonia who fails to respond or who shows predisposing factors.	Blood gases usually show hypoxia and respiratory alkalosis. Chest x-ray may be normal or show areas of atelectasis or hypoperfusion, or may show areas of infarcts. Pleural effusion is common. Pleural tap: frequently bloody effusion. EKG and Echo: evidence of right heart strain. Ventilation-perfusion scan may	Anticoagulation with heparin. Some patients may require embolectomy or insertion of an "umbrella."

ACUTE PNEUMONITIS

		show multiple perfusion defects, but if clinical suspicion is high, angiography should be performed even if V/Q scan is "low-probability."	
2. Pulmonary infiltrate with eosinophila (PIE) syndrome.	Associated with asthma, parasitic infection, or vasculitis. Chronic form is associated with multiple infective agents. Other considerations include: eosinophilic leukemia, Loeffler's endocarditis, Goodpasture's syndrome, lymphomas, sarcoid, tuberculosis, drug reactions, asthma with bronchopulmonary aspergillosis, extrinsic allergic alveolitis, and Wegener's granulomatosis.	Transient infiltrates with peripheral eosinophila. Pulmonary infiltrate that is recurrent may be helpful diagnostic clue. High peripheral eosinophil count. Eosinophils in sputum (Wright's stain). Careful work-up for appropriate parasitic and fungal infections. (see Aspergillus above).	Treat associated disease specifically if indicated. Corticosteroids helpful in some cases.

3

CEREBROSPINAL FLUID PLEOCYTOSIS

An etiologic diagnosis of infections involving the central nervous system (CNS) is important, since many are both life-threatening and treatable. Thus the clinician must have a high index of suspicion of CNS infection, even when the classic symptoms and signs are missing. Furthermore, the etiology of the CNS infection must be determined quickly so that specific therapy can be instituted.

The classic symptoms and signs of CNS infection include fever, headache, meningismus (nuchal rigidity, and Kernig's and Brudzinski's signs), mental changes, and evidence of increased intracranial pressure. Seizures, paresis, and cranial nerve palsies may also be present. Sometimes, however, the findings can be much more subtle. For example, a newborn may be afebrile and reveal only lethargy or behavioral changes with or without a bulging fontanelle and a stiff neck. Also, the elderly patient may present with only fever and personality change or obtundation.

The diagnosis of a CNS infection may also be delayed because of the presence of a confused mental state that may then be erroneously attributed to an underlying illness. Misdiagnosis is particularly common in patients with stroke, diabetes, or alcoholism, in whom cerebral depression is attributed to the underlying diseases, and the associated CNS infection is overlooked.

In evaluation of CNS infection, a lumbar puncture (LP) is of great value. However, the danger of this test must be kept in mind. If there is evidence of a space-occupying lesion, increased intracranial pressure, and no evidence of frank meningitis, a tap should be withheld, since herniation of the brain stem may occur. If papilledema is present, one must be very wary of performing a spinal tap, since this clinical finding is extremely rare in meningitis alone. On the other hand, increased pressure is not a contraindication to the LP if meningitis is strongly suspected, even if evidence for a space-occupying lesion exists. Under the latter circumstances, a small gauge needle should be used and only enough fluid withdrawn to perform the essential laboratory examinations and cultures.

Causes of CNS infection can be grouped according to treatability and by the type of cerebrospinal fluid changes resulting from the infection (Table 3.1).

Treatable causes of CNS infection include meningoencephalitis caused by pyogenic bacteria, tuberculosis, fungal infections, parasitic and spirochetal infections, and viral infection due to herpes simplex and varicella-zoster. Also treatable are parameningeal foci of infection such as cerebral thrombophlebitis, epidural abscess, or brain abscess.

THREE BASIC SETS OF SPINAL FLUID FINDINGS IN CNS INFECTIONS

These treatable infections can produce three basic types of cerebrospinal fluid (CSF) changes (Table 3.2): one type, designated by us as Type A, has a high cell count, in the thousands, with mostly PMLs (polymorphonuclear leukocytes), elevated protein, and a low glucose level. (Low CSF glucose or hypoglycorrhachia is defined as CSF glucose less than 40% of a serum glucose determination obtained 30 minutes before the LP. In practice, however, a simultaneous blood sugar is generally used.) Type B spinal fluid contains a preponderance of PMLs or lymphocytes or a mixture of both, low sugar and high protein levels, and is found particularly in granulomatous and neoplastic meningitis, although these groups of diseases may produce spinal fluid findings resembling any of the three types discussed. Type C spinal fluid has a cell

TABLE 3.1. CEREBROSPINAL FLUID PLEOCYTOSIS

A. Treatable by specific antimicrobial agents
   1. Type A fluid
      a. Bacterial meningitis (pneumococcus, meningococcus, haemophilus, streptococcus, Listeria, etc.)
      b. Ruptured brain abscess
      c. Amebic meningoencephalitis
   2. Type B fluid
      a. Granulomatous meningitis
         1. Tuberculous
         2. Fungal
   3. Type C fluid
      a. Parameningeal infection
         1. Brain abscess
         2. Subdural abscess
         3. Cerebral epidural abscess
         4. Cerebral thrombophlebitis
         5. Spinal epidural abscess
         6. Otitis/sinusitis
         7. Retropharyngeal abscess
      b. Miscellaneous infections
         1. Mycoplasmal infection
         2. Listeria meningitis
         3. Syphilis
         4. Lyme disease
         5. Rickettsial meningitis
         6. Leptospirosis
         7. Cerebral malaria
         8. Trichinosis
         9. Toxoplasmosis
         10. Trypanosomiasis
      c. Toxic encephalopathy (associated with systemic bacterial infection)
      d. Viral infection (herpes simplex I + II, varicella-zoster)

B. Not treatable by specific antimicrobial agents.
   1. Type C fluid
      a. Postinfectious and postvaccinal encephalitis
      b. Viral meningitis (mumps, coxsackie, echovirus, lymphocytic choriomeningitis, arboviruses, and others)

DIFFERENTIAL DIAGNOSIS OF INFECTIOUS DISEASES

TABLE 3.2. DESCRIPTION OF CSF TYPES

Fluid Type	WBC	Predominant Cell Type	Glucose	Protein (mg%)
Normal	< 5	All mononuclear	Normal 40–80 mg % or at least 40% of the simultaneous blood sugar.	< 50 mg %
A	1000–10,000	90% PMLs	Low in most cases	100–700
B	25–500	Mononuclear (PMLs early)	Low, but may be normal	50–500
C	5–1,000	Mononuclear (PMLs early)	Normal, but rarely quite low	< 100

count in the hundreds, with mostly lymphocytes, normal or raised protein level, and a normal glucose level. This last type of CSF is frequently associated with nontreatable viral infection, but, as will be discussed below, the treatable CNS infections produce numerous variations of these "classic" spinal fluids, and treatable diseases may produce CSF of the A, B, or C variety.

It is important to remember that infection may be superimposed on a spinal fluid that is already abnormal for other reasons; this produces a confusing CSF picture. Examples are patients with AIDS (many of whom have a small number of lymphs and elevated protein due to HIV infection alone) and patients with meningeal carcinomatosis.

TREATABLE INFECTIONS WITH TYPE A CSF FINDINGS

Of the treatable infections, Type A CSF is found in bacterial meningitis, ruptured brain abscess, and Naegleria (amebic) meningoencephalitis. It is important to remember that although some processes (e.g., viral meningitis) classically cause predominantly lymphocytic CSF, in the first 24 to 48 hours they may produce mostly PMLs and therefore be confused with Type A. For example, if a young individual who is not terribly ill has a spinal fluid showing fewer than 100 cells, mostly PMLs, and if early viral meningitis is suspected, one can withhold antimicrobial treatment while carefully observing the clinical course. If the patient remains stable, a retap should be done in 8 to 24 hours, and if it shows a shift to the more characteristic mononuclear pleocytosis of viral meningitis (Type C pattern), antibiotic therapy can be avoided. If the patient deteriorates or the retap fails to show a change toward more lymphocytes, therapy must be started.

Common Causes of Bacterial Meningitis

Bacterial meningitis may present with an influenza-like syndrome, with headaches, fever, lethargy, and neck soreness. As the patient's condition worsens and these signs become more pronounced, the indications for an LP become more obvious.

The causative organism can be suspected on the basis of the patient's age. The most likely pathogens are listed below:

1. Newborns: Streptococci, especially group B; Gram-negative rods such as *E. coli*, particularly those with K1 capsular antigen; and *Listeria monocytogenes*.
2. 3 months to 18 years: *H. influenzae*, Pneumococcus, Meningococcus
3. 18 months to 50 years: Meningococcus, Pneumococcus.
4. Over 50: Pneumococcus most likely, occasionally Meningococcus, Gram-negative rods, or *L. monocytogenes*.

Pneumococcal Meningitis

There are some important clues that allow one to suspect the pneumococcus as the cause of a given case of meningitis. For example, the pneumococcus is the usual meningeal pathogen when the disease is secondary to pneumonia, sinusitis, otitis, or mastoiditis. Furthermore, one should suspect pneumococcal meningitis in patients with head trauma, alcoholism, sickle cell anemia, multiple myeloma, or splenectomy. In patients with recurrent meningitis, the pneumococcus is responsible for most instances.

Although the spinal fluid usually is loaded with PMLs and organisms in pneumococcal meningitis, when the infection is discovered very early, the CSF may show numerous organisms but no PMLs. The mortality rate of pneumococcal meningitis remains high (20 to 80 percent), especially in older age groups. This may in part be related to the presence of the cerebral arteritis and brain destruction seen when the pneumococcus infects the meninges. In recent years the pneumococcus has shown increasing resistance to penicillin. Thus, penicillin can no longer be relied upon for initial coverage in many locales, and empiric therapy with cefotaxime or even cefotaxime plus vancomycin is recommended until sensitivity testing is complete.

Meningococcal Meningitis and Meningococcemia

Meningococcal infection causes two important syndromes that overlap considerably. At one end of the spectrum is meningococcal meningitis, a disease that may occur in any age group, but which is found primarily in children or healthy young adults. The disease may be seen either sporadically or in epidemic form in crowded, closed areas such as military bases, nursing homes, or boarding schools. Petechiae are particularly suggestive of meningococcal infection, although they are found in a variety of types of bacterial meningitis. A Gram stain of the petechial lesions may be diagnostic if Gram-negative diplococci are present. Meningococcal meningitis has a mortality of only 5 percent and has the lowest incidence of sequelae among bacterial meningitides. At the other end of the spectrum of meningococcal disease is the syndrome of meningococcemia, which may be fulminant and overwhelming, causing death in a few hours. This syndrome is characterized by the onset of fever, shock, petechiae, and ecchymoses with little evidence of severe meningeal involvement. In fact, the CSF may show organisms but few, if any, PMLs and normal protein and glucose levels in fulminant cases. Immediate recognition and therapy are essential for survival.

Haemophilus influenzae Meningitis

H. influenzae meningitis is seen mainly in the fall and winter, but can occur at any time of the year. The usual primary infection is either a pharyngitis, sinusitis, epiglottitis, or otitis, which may not be recognized. Petechiae are rarely present. *H. influenzae* meningitis is primarily found in young children less than five years of age, although rarely it may occur in adults, especially those with alcoholism or immunoglobulin deficiencies. Mortality is low (5 percent), but morbidity may be striking. Complications include sterile effusions and cortical vein thromboses, which can cause seizures. On Gram stain, the haemophilus is easily misinterpreted by inexperienced observers as a meningococcus, or if incompletely decolonized, as a pneumococcus.

After consideration of the three major bacterial etiologies of meningitis, a variety of other bacteria should be considered, especially in certain settings.

Other Causes of Bacterial Meningitis

Streptococci cause meningitis secondary to sinusitis, otitis, or bacteremia. In infants, group B streptococci are one of the commonest causes of meningeal infection. Enterobacteria and pseudomonads are other important causes of infection in infants; neonatal meningitis is occasionally caused by a combination of streptococci and Gram-negative organisms. *P. aeruginosa* infection has occurred as a complication of LPs performed with contaminated antiseptic solutions, and *K. pneumoniae* infection, although very rare in adults, has been seen in patients with diabetes mellitus who develop bacteremia from a urinary tract infection.

L. monocytogenes usually produces a Type A CSF, but about 20 percent of the time may cause a low CSF cell count, with mostly lymphocytes and a normal glucose level. Listeria should therefore be considered in meningitis where the spinal fluid is primarily Type A or C, especially if the meningeal infection occurs in an infant, an alcoholic, a patient with a neoplasm, or a patient with an immunologic defect, particularly one involving T-lymphocytes.

The organism is a Gram-positive rod and may resemble diphtheroids or pneumococci on Gram stain, but cultures can be distinguished readily in most laboratories by observing the "tumbling motility" characteristic of Listeria. Some studies suggest that the organisms are frequently not seen on Gram stain, even though they can be grown when the CSF is cultured.

It is important to remember that the third-generation cephalosporins are not adequate for Listeral infections, so that if Listeria is possible and a third-generation cephalosporin was selected for therapy, ampicillin or penicillin or Bactrim should be added.

Finally, some patients with bacterial meningitis have anatomic predispositions, such as penetrating trauma or neurosurgery (in which case Staphylococcus and enteric Gram-negative bacilli are frequent causes) or indwelling shunts (often infected by coagulase-negative staphylococci, diphtheroids, and rarely enteric Gram-negative bacilli) and cerebrospinal fluid leaks (usually complicated by pneumococcal infection).

Diagnostic Studies to Detect Specific Etiology of Bacterial Meningitis (Table 3.3)

The bacterial infections discussed above usually have a Type A spinal fluid. Bacteremia is present in about 50 percent of the cases. Cultures of the CSF are positive in about 90 percent. Since the blood culture is occasionally positive when the CSF culture is negative, blood cultures should always be performed in the evaluation of a patient with meningitis. The Gram stain is the most crucial study and is diagnostic in 80 to 90 percent of proven cases. At times the Gram stain may show the organism even when the culture is negative, especially if antibiotics have been given. Other laboratory aids are the methylene blue and acridine orange stains, which may detect the presence of bacteria when the Gram stain shows no organisms. The Quellung reaction, CIE and ELISA may all identify bacterial antigens, and the recently-developed polymerase chain reaction (PCR) shows great promise in the specific identification of nucleic acid, even when organisms are no longer viable.

TABLE 3.3 STUDIES INDICATED FOR EVALUATION OF CSF

Tube	Volume	Studies
Tube 1	1 ml	RBC, WBC, and differential count
Tube 2	1 ml	Protein, glucose (compare with simultaneous blood glucose)
Tube 3	2 ml	Culture → Bacteria (blood agar, chocolate agar, in 10% CO_2 at 37 C) / Fungi (Sabouraud's) / TB (L-J)
Tube 4 (centrifuge 1 ml and sediment)		Gram stain — May do Quellung if antisera is available. Methylene blue stain may be helpful if Gram stain negative. India ink preparation / AFB stain (see text) — If meningitis suspected, but Gram stain negative. Send remainder for VDRL and cryptococcal antigen
Tube 5	1-2 ml	Extra: may need to do viral cultures or other studies. (Request lab save all extra fluid, since more specialized studies may be indicated after initial results are obtained and clinical course is followed.) If indicated: Viral cultures, Wet prep., cresyl fast stain. Additional specialized tests: CIE, limulus test, cytology, ELISA, PCR

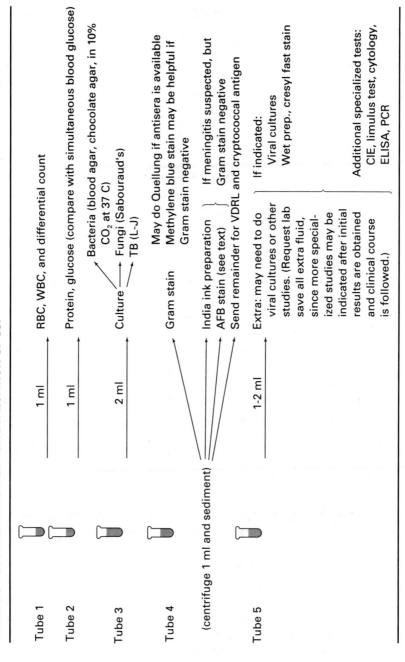

Ruptured Brain Abscess

Meningitis may also be produced when a brain abscess ruptures. In this situation the CSF pressure is usually very high, the cell count over 100,000 with 90 percent PMLs, and the glucose level depressed. An additional clue to a ruptured brain abscess is the presence, in the adult CSF, of a mixture of Gram-positive cocci and Gram-negative rods, especially if anaerobic.

Amebic Meningitis

A third cause of Type A spinal fluid is meningoencephalitis caused by *Naegleria fowleri*. This infection should be suspected when a healthy and active young person with a history of recent swimming in a freshwater lake becomes ill with meningitis and shows a negative CSF Gram stain. In the United States, most cases have occurred in the South (Virginia, Florida, and Texas), but the disease also has been recognized in many other parts of the world. The CSF may show a large number of red, as well as white, cells. For diagnosis, an unstained wet preparation should be examined for motile organisms. A stain of the CSF with cresyl fast violet is particularly helpful in detecting these unusual infecting agents. Cultures of the CSF should be performed in Page's nonnutrient agar. Therapy with amphotericin B should be attempted, although it is not of proven value in vivo. A related amebic infection, caused by Acanthameba, is seen in immunocompromised patients often with associated pulmonary or skin involvement.

TREATABLE INFECTIONS ASSOCIATED WITH TYPE B CSF FINDINGS

Among the causes of Type B spinal fluid, tuberculosis remains an important consideration. Tuberculosis meningitis usually has a subacute onset and progression with 200 to 300 WBCs, mostly lymphocytes. As the disease progresses, the glucose level drops gradually to an extremely low value and the protein level slowly rises. However, on occasion tuberculous meningitis may simulate bacterial meningitis, because it may begin acutely, especially after trauma, and because in the early infection, the CSF may contain mostly PMLs. Furthermore, the cell count may be much greater than the usual 200 to 300 cells/mm^3. On the other hand, there are times when the only CSF abnormality is minimal CSF pleocytosis, which is predominantly lymphocytic (Type C CSF).

Tuberculous meningitis occurs either as part of a primary infection (in younger individuals) or as a result of a reactivation of a latent focus (in older people). The tuberculin skin test is positive in about 80 percent of cases. Although evident in only one-half the cases, extra-neural tuberculosis should be sought elsewhere, especially in the lungs, liver, and bone marrow.

The findings on CSF, though suggestive, are rarely diagnostic, because the acid-fast or fluorochrome stain is usually negative. There are several methods available to increase the yield on acid-fast smears of the CSF:

1. If a pellicle forms in the CSF on standing, it should be stained.
2. High-speed centrifugation should be employed.
3. Sequential drops of CSF sediment should be allowed to dry on a slide, one on top of the other, for about 6 to 8 drops. Then the "stack" of drops may be stained.

However, even with these additional aids, the stain of the CSF is usually negative in most laboratories. The organism is found on culture in about three-fourths of the cases, but it takes 2 to 6 weeks to grow. Therefore, if tuberculous meningitis is suspected, the clinician must institute therapy before results of CSF cultures are available.

Tuberculosis produces a cerebral arteritis, causes severe basilar meningeal involvement and affects cranial nerves. Bilateral sixth nerve palsy with compatible CSF findings is very suggestive of tuberculosis. Tuberculous meningitis leaves psychiatric and/or neurologic sequelae in 25 percent of survivors. The extensive vasculitis produced may be demonstrated by arteriographic studies. Even with appropriate therapy, approximately 25 percent of patients with tuberculous meningitis die.

Fungal Meningitis

Fungal meningitis also characteristically produces Type B CSF findings, but can also cause Type C CSF findings. This form of meningitis is usually caused by *Cryptococcus neoformans* or *Coccidioides immitis*. Histoplasmosis and blastomycosis may also rarely be associated with meningeal syndromes. In a nonendemic area for coccidioidomycosis, the most common cause of fungal meningitis is the cryptococcus. Also, cryptococcal infection is the most common form of meningitis in AIDS (see Chapter 13). The CSF in cryptococcal meningitis resembles that in tuberculous meningitis, and classically both diseases are usually subacute. Occasionally, cryptococcal meningitis may relapse and remit untreated for years. Other than in AIDS, this infection occurs especially in association with diabetes, leukemia, lymphoma, and/or corticosteroid therapy, but also occurs in apparently healthy individuals. Diagnosis of cryptococcal meningitis can be made by India ink preparation; by culture of CSF, blood, and urine; and by cryptococcal antigen determinations on CSF and blood. The presence of rheumatoid factor may produce a false-positive test for cryptococcal antigen in sera but not in spinal fluid. In meningitis the CSF will show cryptococcal antigen in more than 90 percent of cases.

TREATABLE INFECTIONS ASSOCIATED WITH TYPE C CSF FINDINGS

Some treatable causes of meningitis produce Type C CSF findings, characterized by several hundred cells, mostly lymphocytes, with normal or minimally elevated protein and normal glucose levels. Gram stains and routine cultures are negative. This finding gave rise to the term "aseptic meningitis," a designation that is not accurate, since infectious etiologies are usually responsible for the syndrome. Treatable causes of Type C spinal fluid may be produced by (a) partially treated bacterial meningitis (rare), (b) parameningeal foci of infections, (c) a variety of specific infectious agents, and (d) occasional cases of granulomatous meningitis (discussed previously).

Partially Treated Bacterial Meningitis

Partially treated bacterial meningitis may rarely present with Type C CSF findings, so that questions regarding recent antibiotic administration are imperative. However, the vast majority of patients with bacterial meningitis who have received antibiotics before having an LP show the characteristic Type A spinal fluid findings, although Gram stains and cultures may be negative.

Parameningeal Infections

One group of treatable infections that causes meningismus, fever, and Type C CSF findings comprises the parameningeal infections such as brain abscesses, subdural and epidural abscesses, cerebral thrombophlebitis, mastoiditis and sinusitis, and vertebral or cranial osteomyelitis.

Characteristically, a brain abscess is manifested by headaches, mild fever, mental changes, localizing neurologic signs, seizures, lethargy, and obtundation. However, many patients may have only one or two of these symptoms or signs. Therefore, a high index of suspicion is required to diagnose brain abscess. This entity should be suspected in any patient with a known predisposing disease such as pneumonia, empyema, sinusitis, or congenital cyanotic heart disease, if any of the previously mentioned findings is present.

If a brain abscess is strongly suspected, an LP should not be done unless a mass lesion is ruled out by CT scan (with contrast) or MRI. Care should be taken to look for the presence of multiple abscesses, since these are sometimes overlooked when a single, obvious lesion is found. Nearly all brain abscesses are caused by anaerobic cocci or anaerobic Gram-negative rods or aerobic Gram-positive cocci, especially streptococci or staphylococci. Often more than one type of bacteria is involved. The time-honored treatment of brain abscesses requires surgical drainage and antibiotics, although some focal bacterial infections of the brain can resolve without surgical drainage, and are referred to as cerebritis. The entity of abscess, therefore, comprises a spectrum ranging from cerebritis to an encapsulated liquified abscess requiring drainage.

If an LP is performed, the opening pressure is almost always found to be elevated. Although the CSF usually shows a few to several hundred lymphocytes/mm^3, and normal glucose and high protein levels, the findings can be highly variable, e.g., the cell count may be predominantly polymorphonuclear or the CSF findings may be completely normal. The variability in cell count depends on (a) the proximity of the abscess to the ventricles or subarachnoid space and (b) the degree of encapsulation of the abscess, which is directly proportional to its age. If the abscess is more acute, less encapsulated, and closer to the subarachnoid space, Type A CSF findings are more likely to be found.

Subdural empyema follows sinus or ear infection, especially chronic frontal sinusitis. The patient with this disease complains of pain, fever, somnolence, meningismus and shows localizing signs such as seizures, hemiplegia, and hemiparesis resulting from cortical vein phlebitis (50 percent). The best diagnostic tool is MRI and at times, angiography. Therapy includes both drainage and antibiotics.

Cerebral epidural abscess differs from subdural abscess in its paucity of focal signs. It is usually secondary to frontal sinusitis and is therefore caused most often by the pneumococcus and the streptococcus. Important signs are osteomyelitis of the frontal bone, pitting edema of the forehead, and skull tenderness. Suspicion of this entity should be raised when headache and fever persist after treatment of a sinus or ear infection. CSF findings are usually either Type C or normal. MRI is the diagnostic procedure of choice.

Cerebral thrombophlebitis is another cause of meningismus, fever, and Type C CSF. It can involve the superior sagittal sinus (seizures with a septic focus in the head), cavernous sinus (orbital congestion and exophthalmos secondary to suppuration in the orbit or upper face), or lateral sinus (mastoid swelling, jugular vein tenderness, and superficial vein distension secondary to otitis or mastoiditis). Diagnostic aids include CT scan and angiography. Pulmonary emboli may occur, especially from the lateral sinus, and may help suggest this diagnosis. Treatment necessitates antibiotics and surgical drainage of suppurative foci. The effectiveness of anticoagulants in the treatment of cerebral thrombophlebitis is debatable.

On occasion, severe otitis, mastoiditis, sinusitis, and osteomyelitis of the skull may produce a Type C CSF response.

Two other syndromes that may be associated with a Type C CSF response deserve mention. Spinal epidural abscess should be suspected in patients with fever, back pain or tenderness, and signs of spinal cord compression. Usually, however, this triad of findings is not complete on initial presentation, so that the clinician must be alert to this process. An epidural abscess may be posterior, where often it is discovered inadvertently at the time an LP is performed. The most common etiology of a posterior epidural abscess is *S. aureus*, presumably secondary to bacteremia. When a spinal epidural abscess is anterior in location, it is generally secondary to vertebral osteomyelitis, and the bacterial etiology is more variable. In a patient with vertebral osteomyelitis, spinal epidural abscess should be suspected when symptoms of cord compression develop. An x-ray of the spine may detect some soft-tissue abnormalities, but the bony changes of vertebral osteomyelitis are usually found only late in the course of infection. MRI or CT help define the presence and extent of the process, but the specific infectious etiology must be determined by obtaining specimens for stains and cultures at surgery, which should be performed as soon as possible both for its therapeutic effect as well as to allow appropriate antibiotic selection. Surgical drainage must be done immediately to prevent paralysis.

Bacterial endocarditis may produce a sterile CSF pleocytosis along with diffuse encephalopathy, meningismus, or vascular syndromes like hemiplegia. The CSF may be completely normal or show a low cell count with a predominance of either PMLs or lymphocytes and normal sugar values. The fluid is almost always sterile, except in acute endocarditis, when typical purulent meningitis may occur. The combination of pneumococcal pneumonia and meningitis is frequently seen in association with endocarditis, and this triad of events has been known as "Osler's triad."

An encephalopathy may also be present in patients with other acute infectious processes such as bacteremia. This "toxic encephalopathy" is generally of short duration and occurs most frequently in children and in the very old. Fever, confusion, and irritability or somnolence are seen, with or without meningismus. The CSF is sterile, usually with either normal or Type C findings. The symptoms regress after treatment of the underlying infection.

Rarely, a postinfectious encephalitis may occur following viral infections, especially measles and mumps, and after scarlet fever. Encephalopathies sometimes occur after vaccination for smallpox, rabies, pertussis, or yellow fever.

A variety of other treatable infections are associated with Type C spinal fluid. In many areas of the United States, especially the Southeast and Rocky Mountain areas, rickettsial infections such as Rocky Mountain spotted fever (RMSF) must be considered in any patient with severe headache, fever, rash, and myalgias, especially if there has been possible or definite exposure to ticks. The intense headache and fever should lead to an LP, which will usually reveal a minimal increase in WBCs with either a polymorphonuclear or lymphocytic preponderance. The rash of RMSF usually develops 2 to 6 days after the onset of fever, beginning as red maculopapules, and may progress to petechiae over several days involving first the distal extremities, including palms and soles, and then the trunk. In its severe form, RMSF may resemble meningococcemia. Ordinarily, however, the rash in meningococcemia has a variable distribution, develops early in the disease, rapidly becomes petechial or ecchymotic, and may be tender.

Specific Infectious Agents

Syphilitic Meningitis

An acute or subacute meningitis may occur in syphilis a few months to years following the primary infection, but when present is usually detected within one year of exposure. In 10 percent of the cases, the CNS syndrome is seen concomitant with the rash of secondary syphilis. Patients with the secondary form are usually afebrile, and although the meningitis is self-limited, penicillin treatment must be instituted if the incidence of residual cranial nerve palsies or focal cerebral damage caused by the vasculitis is to be reduced. Some AIDS patients with syphilis have low CSF glucose.

Lyme Disease

Another spirochetal disease with neurologic involvement is Lyme disease. Following the cutaneous inoculation of the organism, the large erythematous lesion of erythema chronicum migrans develops. This may be followed by a meningoencephalitis. Cranial nerve palsies (especially C-VII) and radiculitis are additional manifestations of Lyme neurologic disease and are characteristic enough (in combination with meningoencephalitis) to suggest the diagnosis.

Leptospiral Meningitis

Leptospirosis may cause a meningitis along with fever, headache, myalgias, and conjunctival suffusion. Although jaundice is a helpful clue, most patients with leptospirosis are not jaundiced. A history of contact with rodents, dogs, and farm animals or exposure to water contaminated by these animals is helpful. In some cases a typical biphasic illness is present. The first phase consists of fever, chills, myalgias, and headache for 3 to 6 days, during which the organisms are in the blood and CSF. Following an asymptomatic interval of 1 to 3 days, the second phase, the so-called "immune" stage, presents with recurrence of the earlier symptoms plus meningitis and, at times, renal or hepatic dysfunction. Proteinuria is quite common in leptospiral meningitis. The benefit of antibiotics in leptospirosis is questionable, but early therapy with penicillin G or tetracycline is thought by some to reduce the severe complications of hepatic and renal failure.

Malaria

Malaria may be seen in the United States, and falciparum malaria may cause severe CNS complications. Careful questioning of the patient concerning travel to an endemic area or possible exposure to contaminated needles or blood is mandatory. A peripheral blood smear should be done immediately if malaria is suspected. Since falciparum malaria has a high fatality rate, it is urgent that the diagnosis be rapidly made and that the area of the world where the patient became infected be identified, since falciparum malaria is often chloroquine resistant. Vivax malaria parasites rarely cause serious CNS complications and are nearly always susceptible to chloroquine.

Trichinosis

When trichinosis is complicated by meningitis, obvious clues such as peripheral eosinophilia, myalgias, periorbital edema, and splinter or subungual hemorrhages are present. Careful examination of the CSF may reveal the presence of eosinophils and, occasionally, the causative parasite.

Toxoplasmosis

Toxoplasmosis is another potentially treatable disease that produces a Type C spinal fluid. Central nervous system toxoplasmosis may occur as a simple aseptic meningitis in a normal host, as a severe necrotizing encephalitis in an immunocompromised individual, as multiple abscesses in patients with advanced AIDS, or as part of the syndrome of congenital toxoplasmosis. In children with congenital CNS toxoplasmosis, the CSF protein level may be extremely elevated.

Herpes Simplex Type 1, Meningoencephalitis

The infection often presents with fever, mental and emotional changes, seizures, and altered sensorium. The LP usually shows a Type C response, and the EEG and brain scan may show evidence of a focal lesion, most commonly in the frontal or temporal lobes. Direct diagnosis by brain biopsy is the most specific approach, but treatment is often undertaken empirically with Acyclovir, if the presentation is suggestive. Success of therapy, as measured by survival and absence of neurologic sequelae, is dependent upon early institution of therapy. Herpes simplex Type

II may cause a benign meningitis during the course of primary genital infection. This is a *milder* disease than the herpes Type 1 encephalitis.

The related virus, varicella-zoster, may also cause a meningoencephalitis during the course of varicella or zoster that is treatable with Acyclovir. The CSF is usually Type C, also.

Mycoplasma pneumoniae is a treatable infection that may produce a Type C spinal fluid, although occasionally the CSF glucose is low. Mycoplasma causes meningoencephalitis, occasionally with focal signs like CVA or myelitis. Respiratory disease may be absent or may precede or follow the neurologic illness by days or even weeks.

NONTREATABLE INFECTIONS ASSOCIATED WITH TYPE C SPINAL FLUID

At this time no antiviral therapy has been proven to be efficacious for other viral CNS syndromes. These viral infections are usually preceded by systemic symptomatology. Typically, the patient is otherwise in good health and has had a recent onset of headache, photophobia, myalgias, and stiff neck. Fever may be absent and the extreme "toxicity" is rare. When viral infections involve the CNS, the clinical manifestations are predominantly those of either meningitis or encephalitis, depending on the inciting agent.

Though the CSF abnormalities produced by viral infections are primarily of the Type C variety, PMLs may predominate in the CSF early in viral infection as discussed earlier in this chapter.

Occasionally, the CSF glucose level is reduced in viral infection, particularly in infections due to mumps, lymphocytic choriomeningitis (LCM), herpes simplex and varicella-zoster. In AIDS, some patients with CMV also have lowered CSF glucose.

The most common causes of viral meningoencephalitis are enteroviruses and mumps; less frequent causes include arboviruses in some parts of the country, lymphocytic choriomeningitis, influenza, and EB virus. Knowledge of the epidemiology of these infections will frequently suggest the specific viral etiology. For example, in the late winter or spring, mumps is a likely possibility, whereas arbovirus disease or enteroviral infection is commonest in the summer and early fall. Influenza and lymphocytic choriomeningitis occur most commonly in winter months. EB virus infection occurs throughout the year.

The presence of encephalitis in the animal population (especially birds or horses) raises one's suspicion of arbovirus encephalitis. The presence of pleurodynia, herpangina, or myopericardial syndromes in the human community suggests coxsackie or echovirus activity. A history of contact with mice or hamsters suggest the possibility of LCM infection.

Other clinical findings are also helpful in etiologic diagnosis. The presence of parotitis or orchitis suggests mumps, although coxsackie viruses may also produce these findings. A maculopapular or petechial rash is found with some enteroviral meningitides. Acute HIV infection may present as meningoencephalitis associated with a mono-like illness and a maculopapular or urticarial rash. Occasionally, a co-existent Bell's Palsy (which may be bilateral) is a clue to an HIV etiology, although Bell's may also be seen with EBV, herpes simplex, syphilis and Lyme disease. Arbovirus infection is more likely to produce encephalitis than meningitis, with seizures, stupor, coma, and/or focal findings. Polio can produce paralysis, as can other enteroviral infections, especially of the coxsackie B group, but this is a rare event. Although typical Type C findings predominate in LCM infection, an extraordinarily high CSF lymphocyte count is sometimes found (more than 1000 cells/mm^3).

Making a specific etiologic diagnosis is important for preventive medicine in a community. For example, the diagnosis of several cases of poliomyelitis may indicate that polio immunization is lacking in a significant segment of a community and that aggressive immunization efforts need to be employed.

The diagnosis of arbovirus infection in humans may point out the need for widespread vector control, if further cases are to be prevented.

The specific diagnosis depends on viral isolations and serology. CSF, throat, and stool swabs for viral isolation should be obtained, as well as acute and convalescent sera for serology. EB virus serology is sometimes more useful than a Monospot test in CNS infectious mononucleosis.

TABLE 3.4. DIFFERENTIAL DIAGNOSIS OF NONINFECTIOUS CAUSES OF CSF PLEOCYTOSIS

A. Chemical meningitis
  1. Myelography
  2. Spinal anesthesia
  3. Intrathecal medication

B. Vasculitis

C. Subarachnoid hemorrhage (lowers glucose in 25%)

D. Mollaret's syndrome

E. Behcet's syndrome

F. Lead encephalopathy

G. Sarcoid (may produce Type B CSF)

H. Tumor (leukemia most common; glucose can drop to zero)

I. Seizure activity (must diagnose only if other possibilities are ruled out and if pleocytosis is minimal and rapidly clears)

J. Medications: intravenous gamma globulin, NSAIDS, carbamazepine, penicillin, INH, ciprofloxacin, metronidazole, trimethoprim, sulfonamides, TMP-SMZ, OKT3, azathiaprine.

As a final note of caution, it is important to remember that noninfectious illnesses and even medications may cause "aseptic meningitis" (Table 3.4). Medications implicated have included nonsteroidal antiinflammatory drugs (NSAIDS), penicillin, INH, ciprofloxacin, metronidazole, trimethoprim, sulfonamides, TMP-SMX, OKT3, azathiaprine, carbamazepine, and intravenous gamma-globulin. The CSF cell count may be as high as 2000 to 3000, with a predominance of polymorphonuclear leukocytes, normal glucose, and an elevated protein. This syndrome can be confusing in its mimicry of an infectious process, especially when an antibiotic that itself causes meningitis has been administered to a febrile patient.

DIFFERENTIAL DIAGNOSIS OF INFECTIOUS DISEASES

TABLE 3.5. DIAGNOSTIC CHART: CEREBROSPINAL FLUID PLEO-

Disease	CSF Findings			
	WBC/mm^3	Predominant Cell Type	Sugar (mg%)	Protein (mg%)
Normal CSF	<5	Mononuclear.	40–80 or greater than 40% of the simultaneous blood sugar.	50
A. Infectious diseases associated with CSF pleocytosis				
1. Treatable CNS infection				
a. Bacterial meningitis	1000–10,000 or more. In early bacterial meningitis, WBC may be very low or even zero.	90% PMLs.	Low in majority of cases.	100–700

CYTOSIS—SELECTED ETIOLOGIES

Stains & Cultures	General Comments	Initial Therapy (Alternative Rx in Parentheses)
Negative	Newborns may have slightly higher cell counts (up to 30/mm) and variable predominant WBC types.	
Gram stain is positive in 85% of cases. In addition, culture is positive. If Gram stain is negative, try methylene blue or acridine orange stain to demonstrate bacteria.	In addition to CSF, blood cultures needed. Gram stain smears made of skin petechiae and buffy coat. CSF: Quellung and CIE for pneumococcus, meningococcus and H. flu. Latex agglutination for pneumococcus, H. flu, meningococcus, and E. coli. Limulus test for endotoxin: helpful to pick up Gram-neg-meningitis of hemophilus, meningococcal, enterobacterial, or pseudomonal variety. PCR may become more available.	Pneumococcus: cefotaxime + vancomycin pending sensitivity data. Meningococcus, streptococcus: penicillin G (Cefotaxime). *Haemophilus influenzae*: cefotaxime (Bactrim). Gram-negative rod: gentamicin (IV and intrathecal) + ceftazidime. Etiology unknown in newborn: gentamicin + ampicillin or ceftazidime + ampicillin. Etiology unknown in young child or adult: cefotaxime + ampicillin. Children probably benefit from addition of corticosteroids for H. flu. Empiric therapy for post-neurosurgical infection: vancomycin and ceftazidime; shunt infection: vancomycin and rifampin; and CSF-leak-related meningitis: cefotaxime.

(continued)

TABLE 3.5. (continued) DIAGNOSTIC CHART: CEREBROSPINAL

Disease	CSF Findings			
	WBC/mm^3	Predominant Cell Type	Sugar (mg%)	Protein (mg%)
b. Partially treated bacterial meningitis	Usually resembles bacterial, but rarely may be lower.	Usually resembles bacterial, but rarely may have more lymphocytes.	Usually as in bacterial but may be normal.	Usually as in bacterial but may be normal.
c. Listeria meningitis	10–10,000	Usually as in bacterial, but about 20% of cases are predominantly mononuclear.	Low, but may be normal.	50–500
d. Ruptured brain abscess	>10,000	90% PMLs.	Low	100–1000
e. Amebic meningitis	1000–10,000 or more.	PMLs; some RBCs may be present.	Low in most cases.	50–100 or higher.
f. Tuberculous meningitis	25–500	Mononuclear (may show predominantly PMLs early in course).	Low, but early may be normal.	50–500 or greater.
g. Fungal meningitis	25–500	Mononuclear (may show predominantly PMNs early in course).	Low, but may be normal early.	50–500, but may be normal early.

FLUID PLEOCYTOSIS—SELECTED ETIOLOGIES

Stains & Cultures	General Comments	Initial Therapy (Alternative Rx in Parentheses)
Usually negative Gram stain and culture.	As above, CIE, limulus + PCR may prove helpful.	See above for Bacterial.
Gram stain is frequently negative, but may show Gram-positive coccobacillary rods. Culture positive. Be sure all so-called diphtheroids in CSF are not listeria.	About half of these patients have underlying illness such as lymphoma, other tumors, alcoholism.	Ampicillin (Bactrim)
Gram stain: may show Gram-positive cocci and/or Gram-negative rods. Culture aerobically and anaerobically.	Usually catastrophic. Very high mortality.	Cefotaxime and Flagyl.
Negative Gram stain and routine cultures. Wet mount: cresyl fast stain; special culture procedures-discuss with laboratory.	Severe illness with very high mortality. Of cases in US, Virginia and Florida, lakes important sources of Naegleria.	Amphotericin B
Fluorochrome and AFB stains are positive in about 10%. AFB cultures are positive in 75%	Centrifuge and layer drops of sediment for AFB staining to increase yield. Stain pellicle if present. Apply PPD. Chest x-ray. Consider liver or marrow biopsy and culture.	Isoniazid, rifampin, pyrazinamide and ethambutol.
India ink prep; Gram stain. Fungal cultures.	Cryptococcal antigen and antibody should be looked for in CSF, blood and urine. Urine and blood should be cultured for cryptococci. Sputum smears and cultures should be done if chest x-ray abnormal. Fungal serologies for histoplasmosis and coccidioidomycosis.	Amphotericin B. If cryptococcus suspected or found, add 5-fluorocytosine (if patient does not have AIDS). Possible alternatives include Fluconazole for cryptococcus and intraconazole for coccidiodidomycosis.

(continued)

TABLE 3.5. *(continued)* **DIAGNOSTIC CHART: CEREBROSPINAL**

Disease	CSF Findings			
	WBC/mm^3	Predominant Cell Type	Sugar (mg%)	Protein (mg%)
h. Paramenigeal Infection				
1) Brain abscess (not ruptured)	0–200 (extremely variable)	Mononuclear or PMLs	Normal.	Normal to slightly elevated.
2) Subdural empyema	0–500	Mononuclear or PMLs	Normal.	Normal to slightly elevated.
3) Epidural abscess (cerebral)	0–200	Mononuclear or PMLs	Normal.	Normal to slightly elevated.
(spinal)	0–200	Mononuclear or PMLs	Normal.	Normal to slightly elevated.
4) Cerebral thrombophlebitis	0–200	Usually mononuclear.	Normal.	Frequently elevated.
5) Secondary to otitis, sinusitis, or cranial osteomyelitis.	0–50	Usually mononuclear.	Normal.	Slightly elevated.
i. Miscellaneous infections				
1) Mycoplasma	0–300	Mononuclear	Rarely low usually WNL	Slightly elevated.
2) Syphilis	0–300	Mononuclear.	Normal (may be ↓ in AIDS)	Normal to increased.

FLUID PLEOCYTOSIS—SELECTED ETIOLOGIES

Stains & Cultures	General Comments	Initial Therapy (Alternative Rx in Parentheses)
Negative Gram stain and culture.	MRI, CT scan helpful. Blood cultures should be performed.	Flagyl and cefotaxime ± surgery.
Negative Gram stain and culture.	Diagnostic aids include MRI and angiography. Sinus x-rays are indicated.	Penicillinase-resistant antistaphylococcal penicillin and surgery.[a]
Negative Gram stain and culture.	Skull and sinus x-rays, MRI	Penicillinase-resistant antistaphylococcal penicillin[a] and drainage.
Negative Gram stain and culture.	MRI	Posterior: Penicillinase-resistant antistaphylococcal penicillin + gentamicin or tobramycin or amikacin + drainage.[a]
Negative Gram stain and culture.	MRI, discuss with Radiologist.	Penicillinase-resistant antistaphylococcal penicillin;[a] surgical drainage sometimes indicated. Anticoagulant use is controversial.
Negative Gram stain and culture.	Skull and sinus x-rays may be helpful diagnostically. Other studies as mentioned for brain abscess, especially MRI.	If present, necrotic bone should be removed surgically. Unasyn.
Negative	Cold agglutins, CF serology.	Erythromycin (doxycycline).
Negative Gram stain and culture.	VDRL and FTA-ABS on serum. VDRL on CSF considered diagnostic but not always positive. PCR and antibody production in CSF helpful but not generally available.	Penicillin G.

(continued)

TABLE 3.5. (continued) DIAGNOSTIC CHART: CEREBROSPINAL

Disease	CSF Findings		
	WBC/mm³	Predominant Cell Type	Sugar (mg%)	Protein (mg%)
3) Rocky Mountain Spotted Fever	0–200	Mononuclear or PMNs.	Normal	Normal to slightly elevated.
4) Lyme Disease	0–200	Mononuclear	Normal	Normal to slightly elevated.
5) Leptospirosis	10–500	Mononuclear, occasionally PMNs	Normal	Normal to slightly elevated.
6) Cerebral malaria	0–500	Mononuclear.	Normal.	Normal to slightly elevated.
7) Trichinosis	0–500	Mononuclear or may see eosinophils.	Normal.	Normal to slightly elevated.
8) Toxoplasmosis	100–3000	Mononuclear.	Normal.	Normal or slightly elevated. In children with congenital disease, protein may be very high (1000–2000).

FLUID PLEOCYTOSIS—SELECTED ETIOLOGIES

Stains & Cultures	General Comments	Initial Therapy (Alternative Rx in Parentheses)
Negative Gram stain and bacterial cultures.	Specific rickettsial serologies, PCR if available. Biopsy and stain rash for rickettsia with fluorescent antibody if available. (Tick bite history, rash, clinical course very characteristic. Most cases occur April–September.)	Doxycycline (chloramphenicol).
Negative stain and culture.	Serology usually ⊕.	Ceftriaxone.
Negative stain and culture.	Serology; culture blood, CSF + urine. Need special media.	Value questionable. Penicillin G may reduce hepatic and renal complications if given early.
Negative stain and culture.	Peripheral blood smear (thick and thin).	Chloroquine. If chloroquine resistance suspected, quinine + tetracycline. If parenteral therapy needed, use IV quinidine for quinine.
Negative Gram stain and culture.	Serology and skin test. Muscle biopsy.	Corticosteroids + thiabendazole.
Negative Gram stain and culture. Wright's or Giemsa stain of CSF.	Biopsy of lymph node may show characteristic pathology. Serology.	Pyramethamine + sulfadiazine.

(continued)

DIFFERENTIAL DIAGNOSIS OF INFECTIOUS DISEASES

TABLE 3.5. *(continued)* **DIAGNOSTIC CHART: CEREBROSPINAL**

Disease	CSF Findings			
	WBC/mm³	Predominant Cell Type	Sugar (mg%)	Protein (mg%)
j. Toxic Encephalopathy				
1) Toxic encephalopathy (nonspecific)	0–100	Mononuclear.	Normal.	< 50
2) Bacterial endocarditis	< 500	Mononuclear or PMNs	Normal	50–100
k. Viral infection				
1) Herpes simplex Type I	0–500	Mononuclear	Normal (rarely low)	Normal or elevated.
2) Herpes simplex Type II	0–500	Mononuclear	Normal (rarely low)	Normal to slightly elevated.
3) Varicella-zoster	0–500	Mononuclear	Rarely low	Normal to slightly elevated.
2. Nontreatable CNS infection				
a. Viral meningitis (other than herpes & varicella)	5–1000	Mononuclear (in early phase PMNs may predominate).	Normal (occasionally decreased with LCM, mumps)	Normal or slightly elevated.
b. Postinfectious, postvaccinal	0–100	Mononuclear.	Normal.	Normal to slightly increased.

DIAGNOSTIC CHART: CEREBROSPINAL

Stains & Cultures	General Comments	Initial Therapy (Alternative Rx in Parentheses)
Negative Gram stain and culture.	Workup underlying infectious process.	Therapy directed toward primary infectious process (e.g., Gram-negative bacteremia).
Gram stain and culture are almost always negative.	Blood cultures diagnostic in about 85% of cases.	Acute: Nafcillin (or vancomycin) + gentamicin. Subacute: ampicillin + gentamicin. Prosthetic value: vancomycin + gentamicin ± rifampin.
Can attempt specific viral cultures of CSF, but yield in this infection is low.	Diagnosis usually made clinically or by brain biopsy, with stains and viral cultures. Nonspecific diagnostic aids include CAT scan, EEG, MRI. PCR may prove useful.	Acyclovir
Viral isolation	Mild disease. Seen during primary genital herpes infection.	Acyclovir
Viral isolation.	May precede, accompany or follow varicella-zoster infection. Delayed CNS presentations may be on an immunologic basis. Zoster ophthalmicus sometimes ass'd with contra-lateral hemiplegia.	Acyclovir
Viral cultures of CSF; specific immunofluorescent stain on CSF leukocytes may be useful. Gram stain and bacterial cultures are negative.	Viral cultures should be performed on pharyngeal washings and rectal swabs or any vesicular lesions. Serology also helpful.	No specific therapy.
Negative Gram stain and culture.	History important in suggesting this etiology.	No specific therapy; corticosteroids may be useful.

(continued)

TABLE 3.5. *(continued)* **DIAGNOSTIC CHART: CEREBROSPINAL**

Disease	CSF Findings			
	WBC/mm³	Predominant Cell Type	Sugar (mg%)	Protein (mg%)
B. Noninfectious diseases associated with CSF pleocytosis				
1. Tumor	0–300	Mononuclear and/or tumor cells.	Normal or may be decreased to very low levels.	50 > 1000
2. SLE	< 50	Mononuclear.	Normal.	Normal or slightly elevated.
3. Seizure activity	20	Mononuclear.	Normal.	Normal or elevated.
4. Chemical (myelography dye, intrathecal drugs, ruptured cyst)	100–1000	PMLs.	Normal or low.	Normal or slightly elevated.
5. Molleret's syndrome	500–15,000	PMLs.	Normal.	Normal or slightly elevated.
6. Behcet's syndrome	< 100 usually (may go to 1000)	PMLs or mononuclear.	Normal.	Normal or slightly elevated.
7. Sarcoidosis	0–100	Mononuclear.	Normal to very low.	50–1000
8. Medication	0–3000	PMLs	Normal.	Slightly elevated.

[a] Clinical clues and Gram stain of pus obtained at surgery may dictate alternative antibiotic choices.

FLUID PLEOCYTOSIS—SELECTED ETIOLOGIES

Stains & Cultures	General Comments	Initial Therapy (Alternative Rx in Parentheses)
Negative Gram stain and culture.	Cytologic evaluation of CSF cells may prove diagnosis.	No antimicrobial therapy. Therapy is directed against the particular neoplasm.
Negative Gram stain and culture.	Other criteria for diagnosis of SLE should be present.	Corticosteroids and/or other immunosuppressive agents.
Negative Gram stain and culture.	Must rule out treatable causes before assuming pleocytosis to be associated with seizure activity.	Control of seizure; treatment of underlying cause for seizure.
Negative Gram stain and culture.	Keratin may be noted in polarized light with dermoid cyst.	For most, no specific treatment.
Negative Gram stain and culture.	Stain with H & E—may see endothelial cells. Recurrent process.	No specific therapy.
Negative Gram stain and culture.	History and physical exam demonstrate involvement of other organs such as the eye, GI tract, and mucous membranes.	No specific therapy, but corticosteroids sometimes used.
Negative Gram stain and culture.	Chest x-ray, liver function tests; lymph node and liver biopsy may be helpful, Kveim test, ACE; Gallium Scan.	Corticosteroids.
Negative Gram stain and culture.	Check medications (see text).	Discontinue offending medication.

4

BACTERIURIA AND PYURIA

Among diseases in the United States caused by infectious agents, urinary tract infection (UTI) is second in frequency only to upper respiratory tract disease. Patients with UTIs may have characteristic symptoms or may be asymptomatic, in which case examination of the urine is the first clue to UTI.

SYMPTOMATOLOGY

The genitourinary (GU) tract may be infected from the urethra to the kidney, and the actual site of the infection may be suggested by the type of symptomatology. For example, burning on urination, difficulty in initiating urination, and a urethral discharge suggest urethral inflammation, although infections above the urethra, i.e., in the bladder, ureter, or kidney may also produce these symptoms. With cystitis (bladder inflammation), nocturia, urgency, and pain in the perineal, suprapubic or lumbar areas is frequent.

When symptomatic prostatic inflammation is present, pain in the rectum, back, thighs, perineum and genitalia occurs in addition to symptoms of cystitis and urethritis. Involvement of the renal parenchyma (pyelonephritis) may produce pain the flank and abdomen in addition to symptoms of cystitis and urethritis.

However, such symptomatology is by no means always accurate in this localization of infection. For example, a bacterial cystitis may produce symptoms referable to the kidney, and vice versa. For this reason, some clinicians group these disorders as UTIs "with lower tract symptoms" or "with upper tract symptoms."

LABORATORY TESTS

In evaluating a patient for a UTI, the most important laboratory test is examination and culture of the urine and/or urethral and prostatic discharge. Collection of the urine is important. In females the specimen should be "clean-caught." While sitting comfortably, the patient should be instructed to spread her labia and to wash the urethral area from front to back, rinse, and then collect a midstream specimen. The collection process in males is more reliable, since there is less chance of contamination of the urine. The patient should be instructed to wash the penis (after retracting the foreskin if uncircumcised) and to collect a midstream specimen.

When a patient has an indwelling catheter, urine may be aspirated for examination and culture by the following technique: the catheter near the junction with the drainage tube is prepared as a site for intravenous injection. Then the aspirating needle is introduced at a slant, which guarantees self-sealing of the catheter after removal of the needle. Care should be taken not to force any urine back into the bladder. At no time should a closed drainage system be disconnected to obtain cultures.

The urine specimen should be refrigerated immediately if it is not taken directly to the laboratory, because the organisms will double in number every 30 minutes and make the colony count falsely high and valueless.

If the colony count is greater than 100,000/ml on at least two clean-voided specimens, or on a single urethral catherization, then the patient is considered to have an infection in his bladder or upper urinary tract.

Some infections are associated with lower colony counts, but contamination is an additional consideration with the lower counts. In general, counts lower than 10^5 should be considered as possibly indicative of infection, especially if symptoms or pyuria are present; explanation for the lower counts include overhydration (and consequent dilution), prior antibiotic therapy, and the presence of less usual pathogens such as staphylococci, yeast or chlamydia.

Sometimes suprapubic puncture or urethral catherization may help document an infection with small numbers of bacteria. These procedures are uncomfortable, but in certain patients may be the only means of obtaining a reliable specimen.

The unspun urine should be Gram stained, and the urine sediment should be examined for WBCs. If any bacteria are present on a Gram stain of properly collected, unspun urine, infection is almost certainly present, as this finding correlates well with the presence of a colony count greater than 10^5, the number of organisms found to represent significant infection of the urinary tract. The leukocyte esterase dipstick is a helpful screening procedure and identifies the presence of leukocytes. Similarly, the nitrite reduction test screens urine samples for bacteria.

It may be advantageous to identify those bacteriuric patients with infection localized to the kidney or to the bladder. If those with kidney infection are more likely to develop chronic renal disease, then the subpopulation with bacteriuria localized to the kidney may deserve more intensive medical therapy. To this end, many procedures have been developed to distinguish patients with upper versus lower tract infection. Such methods include the following:

1. Search for the presence of WBC casts in the urine. If WBC casts are found, involvement of the upper urinary tract is strongly suggested.
2. Bladder catheterization with cultures, followed by a washout of the bladder with an antibiotic solution, followed in turn by bilateral urethral catheterization with cultures. This technique is not simple, is expensive, and has hazards. It is impractical and probably dangerous to perform on a large scale.
3. Bladder catheterization with cultures followed by washout to eliminate bladder bacteriuria and then collection of bladder rinse specimens, which now represent bacteria coming from the upper tract. This is simpler than the previous method. Unfortunately, this technique still requires instrumentation, is time-consuming, and fails to distinguish between involvement of one or both kidneys.

4. Fluorescent antiglobulin staining of urine bacteria. Bacteria originating from the upper tract (kidney) or prostate are coated with antibody while those originating from the bladder are not. Thus a urine smear showing antibody-coated bacteria suggests either prostate or upper tract infection.
5. The differentiation between relapse (recurrence due to the same organism) and reinfection (recurrence with a new species or strain of bacteria). Relapse suggests the presence of upper tract infection; reinfection suggests lower tract disease.
6. Radionuclide scanning can identify areas of active infection in the kidney. However, determination of a "complicated" versus "uncomplicated" infection actually provides more prognostic information; thus, infections "complicated" by anatomic abnormalities (obstruction, stone, catheter, etc.) or functional derangement (sickle cell anemia, diabetes) are more difficult to eradicate and are more likely to result in renal damage and septicemia.

The presence of pyuria in clean-caught urine indicates inflammation, infection, or tissue destruction somewhere in the genitourinary tract, from the urethra to the kidneys. By far the most frequent cause of pyuria is bacterial infection of the urethra, bladder, and/or kidneys. The presence of WBC casts strongly suggests renal parenchymal involvement. One must be careful of relying too heavily on the mere presence of WBCs in a urine sediment to diagnose a UTI. In women with cervicitis (usually caused by *N. gonorrhoeae* or *Chlamydia trachomatis*) or vaginitis (usually caused by Trichomonas or Candida) or vaginosis (caused by Gardnerella and other bacteria) WBCs from the vaginal or cervical secretions may contaminate clean-caught urine and thus confuse the diagnosis. Similarly, in the male, balanitis may produce a pyuria without indicating UTI. Furthermore, the absence of pyuria does not rule out the presence of UTI, since significant bacteriuria may occur without pyuria.

Smear and culture of prostatic secretion is helpful in evaluating a patient with possible prostatitis, although prostatic massage should probably be avoided if the prostate is acutely inflamed.

In the following discussion, infections of the GU tract are categorized according to the anatomic area of involvement (Table 4.1).

TABLE 4.1. BACTERIURIA AND PYURIA

A. Urethritis
 1. Gonococcus
 2. Secondary to cystitis or pyelonephritis
 3. Non-gonococcal urethritis (NGU)
 4. Trichomonas
 5. Candida

B. Prostatitis
 1. Acute
 2. Prostatic abscess
 3. Chronic
 4. Non-bacterial prostatitis

C. Cystitis
 1. Bacteria
 2. Candida
 3. *M. tuberculosis*
 4. *Schistosoma hematobium*

D. Pyelonephritis
 1. Bacteria
 2. Candida
 3. *M. tuberculosis*

E. Renal abscess

F. Perinephric abscess

G. Papillary necrosis

H. Abscess encroaching on bladder or urethra, such as appendicular, pelvic, peri-colonic, psoas

I. Asymptomatic bacteriuria

Urethritis

Inflammation of the urethra produces dysuria, difficulty in urinating, and urethral discharge. When these symptoms are present, one cause may be gonorrhea. In the male the diagnosis is established if Gram-negative diplococci with PMLs are seen on the Gram stain of the urethral discharge, and proof by culture is not necessary. In males a urethral discharge should be cultured only if the Gram stain fails to reveal cell-associated Gram-negative diplococci. In females, cultures of the urethra, cervix, and rectum should always be taken, since Gram stains are less reliable for the diagnosis of gonococcal infection.

In the absence of finding gonococci, other causes must be suspected. Candida and trichomonads are sometimes responsible. Diagnosis of candidal urethritis is made via Gram stains of the discharge or by mixing a drop of KOH with the discharge, warming, and examining under a microscope. Trichomoniasis is a sexually transmitted disease that usually is associated with vaginitis in women and prostatitis in men. Diagnosis is made by visualization of the motile parasites on a wet mount, which is prepared by mixing urine or a urethral discharge with a drop of saline and examining the drop immediately under the microscope. If the results of these studies are negative, but there are a significant number of WBCs, then the syndrome of non-gonococcal urethritis (NGU) must be considered. NGU is an extremely common cause of urethritis in males. It is characterized by a slight amount of mucoid discharge or dysuria. Unlike gonococcal urethritis, spontaneous, grossly purulent discharge is rarely seen. NGU is usually caused by *Chlamydia trachomatis*, though some cases are caused by *Ureaplasma urealyticum* and herpes simplex; a significant proportion of cases of NGU have no known etiology.

When urethritis persists and no pathogen can be elucidated, one should consider neurosis on the part of the patient; on occasion, extreme concern over a urethral exudate results in men constantly "milking" their urethra. Such trauma can be itself cause a constant discharge and dysuria. Infective urethritis is not likely if a smear of urethral exudate or a urethral swab fails to show 4 to 5 WBCs per high-power field; similarly, the first 10 cc of voided urine usually contains 10 to 15 WBCs per mm^3 in the presence of urethritis.

Prostatitis

Acute Form

In acute prostatitis, symptoms of urethritis may be present along with pain in the lower back, rectum, or perineum and may radiate to the thighs and genitalia. High fever and chills are sometimes present. The prostate is tense or boggy and very tender. Acute prostatitis is usually an ascending infection, but it may result from hematogenous spread. Predisposing factors are said to include alcoholism, perineal trauma, and excessive sexual activity. Etiologic diagnosis is made by culture and Gram stain of the urine and prostatic secretions, although massage of an acutely inflamed prostate is to be avoided. Blood cultures may occasionally be positive and reveal the specific etiologic agent present. The organisms usually involved in bacterial prostatitis are aerobic Gram-negative rods, especially *E. coli,* and enterococci. *M. tuberculosis* may involve the prostate, but it generally remains asymptomatic.

Prostatitis may be complicated by epididymitis. Epididymitis causes a painful swelling of the scrotum, often with accompanying swelling of the ipsilateral testis, called epididymo-orchitis. Although in young men epididymitis is sexually transmitted and thus caused by gonococcal or chlamydial infection, in men over the age of 35 Gram-negative pathogens causing prostatitis and associated urinary tract infection are the usual etiology of epididymitis.

As opposed to epididymo-orchitis, simple orchitis is usually part of a systemic infection, particularly with mumps or Coxsackie virus.

Prostatic Abscess

Acute prostatitis may develop into a prostatic abscess. This entity should be suspected (a) when an acute bout of prostatic infection fails to respond to therapy within 5 to 7 days, (b) if a fluctuant area is palpated on prostatic examination, or (c) if the patient suffers a relapse after a course of appropriate antimicrobial therapy.

Chronic Form

Unresolved attacks may result in chronic prostatitis manifested by chronic lower lumbar and perineal pain, dysuria, and difficulty urinating. Prostatic examination may be normal, but prostatic secretions contain many WBCs, and bacteria are present in the prostatic discharge and in the urine.

Nonbacterial Prostatitis

Nonbacterial prostatitis is the most common prostatitis syndrome and is manifested by prostatic symptoms, inflammatory cells in prostate secretions, but negative cultures. Etiology is either a chemical inflammation (possibly due to reflux of urine) or infection due to organisms such as chlamydia, mycoplasmas and ureaplasmas.

Prostatodynia

Prostatodynia represents a prostatic pain syndrome but with negative cultures and normal prostatic secretions. This syndrome has been variously attributed to functional obstruction of prostatic secretions, pelvic myalgia, and psychosexual dysfunction.

Cystitis

Cystitis is suggested by dysuria, frequency, nocturia, urgency, and pain or tenderness in perineal, suprapubic, or lumbar areas. It is nearly always caused by bacterial infection, the organism having gained entry to the bladder via the urethra. Cystitis is seen most commonly in women of all ages and in men over the age of 50. Females are more prone than males to bacterial infection of the GU tract because of their shorter urethra, relaxation of the pelvic floor with age and childbearing, and lack of the antibacterial properties of prostatic fluids. Also, in females, sexual intercourse is associated with the movement of urethral bacteria into the bladder. Factors that predispose to cystitis are obstruction, diabetes, catheterization, instrumentation, pregnancy, and neurologic deficit.

There is usually minimal or no fever associated with cystitis. An "uncomplicated" first infection is usually caused by *E. coli*, which is sensitive to most antimicrobial agents, including sulfonamides, ampicillin, and tetracycline. Recurrent infection or infection associated with obstruction or instrumentation, though still most commonly caused by *E. coli*, is sometimes caused by Klebsiella, enterobacter, Proteus, enterococci, and pseudomonads. In this latter group of "complicated infections," the organisms, including even *E. coli*, are frequently resistant to sulfonamides, ampicillin, and tetracycline. Rarely are staphylococci responsible for cystitis. Anaerobic infection of the bladder is distinctly unusual.

C. albicans is occasionally a cause of cystitis, especially in patients with indwelling urinary catheters and those receiving antibiotics and/or corticosteroids. Unfortunately, it is difficult to determine the significance of Candida found on Gram stain or culture of the urine. The significance of colony counts is not as clear as with bacterial infection. Thus more information is required to interpret the presence of persistent Candida in a urine specimen after predisposing factors have been eliminated. Cystoscopy, intravenous pyelogram (IVP), and/or isolation of the organism from urine obtained by suprapubic puncture can assist in differentiating mere colonization from invasive localized candidiasis. With attention to predisposing factors, such as removal of a urinary catheter, discontinuing antibiotics, and treating vaginal and gastrointestinal candidal infection, the urinary Candida colonization usually disappears.

Although candiduria usually represents an ascending infection, it is consistently present as part of the entity of disseminated candidiasis. Thus in the appropriate clinical setting (e.g., immunosuppression, multiple prior antibiotics), the patient with Candida in the urine should be evaluated for evidence of systemic candidiasis.

Signs and symptoms of cystitis may also be caused by tuberculosis. This disorder should be suspected when pyuria is present despite sterile urine. Tuberculous involvement of the lower GU tract always results from tuberculosis in the kidney, which in this country results from the bacillemia associated with primary pulmonary infection. Patients with GU tuberculosis present with symptoms of cystitis or pyelonephritis, sometimes with primarily pulmonary symptoms, and occasionally with constitutional complaints. One half of patients exhibit no evidence of pulmonary disease. Diagnosis is proven by culture of the urine (positive in 80 percent) and sputum (positive in 40 percent) and is suggested by (a) pyuria without bacteriuria, (b) hematuria, (c) positive skin test, and/or (d) cystoscopic findings. The presence of calcifications in the kidney, seminal vesicles, and prostate is suggestive. IVP changes are frequent and may be characteristic.

Kidney Infections

Acute Pyelonephritis

Acute pyelonephritis usually results from bacteria ascending from the bladder. It affects the same age group and has the same etiologies as bacterial cystitis. The tendency for infection of the bladder to localize to the kidney parenchyma is abetted by obstruction and by pre-existing renal damage, particularly in the medulla, which occurs as a result of diabetes, gout, hypertension, analgesic and anti-inflammatory medications, hypercalcemia, and hypokalemia. A damaged medulla is susceptible to pyelonephritis. Pyelonephritis is suggested by fever, chills, prostration, and pain and tenderness in the flank, epigastrium, costovertebral angle, and lumbar area. Infants with pyelonephritis may simply "fail to thrive," and older children may manifest their infection by enuresis and incontinence during the day. Rarely, acute pyelonephritis may produce minimal or no symptoms.

Candida and other fungi may also cause pyelonephritis; signs and symptoms are the same as for bacterial disease. Fungal pyelonephritis is associated with catheters, antibiotics, steroids, GU tract surgery, and underlying renal disease. Occasionally, an IVP may demonstrate abnormalities of the collecting system or the kidney, and actual fungus balls may be passed. Although usually an ascending infection, candidal pyelonephritis may be hematogenous.

GU tuberculosis may present with signs and symptoms of pyelonephritis; diagnosis is established as discussed under tuberculous cystitis.

Renal Abscess

The signs and symptoms described for pyelonephritis may also be seen in the case of a renal abscess. This entity may result from staphylococcal bacteremia, in which case it usually initally involves the renal cortex. In the early phases of cortical abscess, the Gram stain and culture of the urine may be negative or may reveal Gram-positive cocci, but few or no WBCs are seen. When a renal abscess is the result of an unchecked pyelonephritis, the renal medulla is involved and the urine contains Gram-negative bacilli and WBCs. This entity should be suspected when acute pyelonephritis relapses or fails to respond to antibacterial treatment.

These abscesses may develop into an intrarenal carbuncle, drain spontaneously into the renal pelvis, cause a secondary pyelonephritis, and/or rupture into the perirenal space to produce a perinephric abscess. CT scans and sonography are frequently diagnostic.

Perinephric Abscess

Perinephric abscess resembles pyelonephritis clinically, but is more subdued and protracted. The clinical course of perinephric abscess tends to be insidious, and although fever, dysuria, and flank pain are usually present, chills and abdominal pain are not always found. A mass or tenderness in the flank may be detectable. This entity is caused by an extension of pyelonephritis in two-thirds of cases or by staphylococcal bacteremia in one-third. Most patients have either diabetes or renal calculi as the underlying illness. Urinalysis generally demonstrates pyuria, significant proteinuria, and occasionally red blood cells (RBCs). Blood cultures are positive in 40 percent and urine cultures in 70 percent of patients with this entity. Sonography and CT allow both delineation of a mass and evaluation of renal movement.

Other Infections

Papillary Necrosis

Papillary necrosis is a serious clinical problem frequently associated with infection with or without obstruction. The patient may initially appear to have pyelonephritis and renal failure. Instead of responding to antimicrobial treatment, extreme kidney tenderness develops, as well as persistent heavy pyuria and hematuria. As the necrotic papilla is passed, colic may supervene. The picture may be less dramatic, i.e., recurrent bouts of infection and the passage of fragments in the urine, but death from uremia or septicemia is a constant threat.

Papillary necrosis should be suspected in patients with diabetes, interstitial nephritis, analgesic abuse, and sickle cell disease. The disorder is usually seen in patients over the age of 40. Diagnosis is made by finding WBCs, RBCs, bacteria, and tissue fragments in the urine, and deformed papillae on IVP or CT scan.

Abscesses Outside the GU Tract

Rarely, massive pyuria may occur secondary to abscesses outside the genitourinary tract that abut the bladder or urethra and may leak into them. Thus abscesses of the appendix or pelvis, pericolonic area and psoas muscle are considerations in the differential diagnosis of pyuria. Frequently other clinical clues are present to suggest one of these entities. For example, appendiceal abscess may follow an illness in a young patient suggestive of appendicitis, with right lower quadrant pain. Pericolonic abscess is more likely in older patients with diverticulitis, usually producing left lower quadrant symptomatology. Psoas abscess may complicate bacteremia or spread from contiguous infection in the vertebral column, characteristically causing pain that radiates to the inner thigh. Pelvic abscess typically results from gonococcal or non-gonococcal pelvic inflammatory disease, seen in sexually active women with fever, cervical discharge as well as pyuria, and tenderness on physical examination, particularly in the adnexal areas.

Occasionally, a patient will excrete a large amount of pus, but only intermittently, and in these cases one must consider an infected bladder diverticulum, vesicocolonic or vesicovaginal fistula, or pyonephrosis with intermittent obstruction.

Asymptomatic Bacteriuria

Up to this point, the discussion has considered symptomatic disease. However, there exists a group of patients who have a chronic bacteriuria with minimal symptoms known as "asymptomatic bacteriuria," an entity that is not well understood. The best-studied subgroup of patients with asymptomatic bacteriuria consists of pregnant women. If untreated, they are very likely to develop symptomatic disease later in their pregnancy. When symptomatic UTI occurs during pregnancy, fetal wastage may occur. Thus, pregnant patients should be screened for bacteriuria and, if it is present, it should be treated even in the absence of symptoms.

No other subgroup of patients has been shown to benefit from treatment of asymptomatic bacteriuria, although it is felt by some that treatment may at times be indicated for the condition in diabetes, in the elderly, and in "complicated" infection.

MANAGEMENT OF UTI

The treatment of patients with UTI may include urologic evaluation as well as medical therapy. Urologic investigation is indicated in patients who are likely to have correctable obstructing lesions, i.e., (a) neonates, (b) young children of both sexes, (c) all males, and (d) girls and women with frequent infections. Initial workup should include renal and bladder ultrasound; following investigations with CT, IVP and cystoscopy are reserved for special problems and are individualized.

The choice of medical treatment of UTI is dependent not only on the type of bacterium suspected or isolated, but also on host factors and the sites of infection. Acute symptomatic UTI that is "uncomplicated" (not associated with obstruction, stones, or prior infection) is caused by *E. coli* in 85 percent of cases and responds well to a wide variety of antimicrobial drugs of low toxicity. If the infection is "complicated," a situation encountered especially among children and adult males, organisms other than *E. coli*, such as Proteus, Klebsiella, and enterococcus must be considered as well, and the selection of antimicrobial therapy should take this into account. Treatment of the patient with complicated infection must also include a search for surgically-correctable obstructing lesions.

If the patient with acute infection is seriously ill and bacteremia is suspected, the initial regimen chosen should be active against most enterobacteria, pseudomonads, and enterococci (e.g., ampicillin and gentamicin), even if the infection is uncomplicated. The initial therapy of the seriously ill patient with UTI should be parenteral.

If the patient is not ill and appears to have an uncomplicated lower tract infection (e.g., simple cystitis), then a single-dose or (preferably) three-day regimen will often be sufficient. Regimens used for this are predominantly Bactrim or Augmentin.

It is imperative to reculture the urine of patients treated for UTIs, even after apparent symptomatic cure, since bacteriuria may persist in spite of reduction or elimination of symptoms. Infection present after supposed cure is either a relapse or reinfection, and such infection may or may not be symptomatic. Relapse represents persistent infection due to the same organism that caused the previous infection, while reinfection is caused by a different pathogen.

When a patient's recurrent infection is due to reinfection, most clinicians agree that a short course of therapy is as likely to eradicate the bacteria as is a longer course. With relapse, a 6-week course of therapy may be able to eradicate bacteria in some patients who fail to respond to a shorter course of treatment. Most recurrences in men result from relapse, from a focus of infection in the kidney or prostate. On the other hand, most recurrences in women are reinfections, i.e., invasion by a new species or strain of bacterium. When correctable lesions have been eliminated and a patient continues to suffer relapsing infection after a 6-week course, some clinicians advise a trial of long-term (e.g., 6 months) therapy in selected patients, especially children, adults with symptoms and patients with obstructing lesions (because of the risk of renal damage). Women with frequent reinfections often take prophylactic medication before or after coitus. Such regimens may decrease the incidence of symptomatic recurrence in these patients, but their effect on any chronic kidney damage that may result from recurrent infection is unknown.

If a patient is found to have bacteriuria on routine urine culture and is asymptomatic, repeat urine cultures are indicated to be certain contamination is not occurring. If bacteriuria is truly present and fails to respond to a course of antimicrobial therapy, urologic investigation should be initiated with sonography. Unfortunately, if no correctable lesion is found, the bacteriuria may be difficult to eradicate in this group of patients. Therefore, in elderly patients, the risk of superinfection and drug toxicity may outweigh the benefit of repeated or long-term courses of antimicrobial agents. In younger individuals, especially pregnant patients, more aggressive efforts to eradicate or suppress the bacteriuria are indicated.

The antibiotic treatment of prostatitis has been improved with the development of agents that penetrate glandular tissue well, e.g., TMP-SMX and the quinolones.

Candida infection of the bladder and kidney is difficult to treat. Pyelonephritis, as a parenchymal infection, is treated with IV amphotericin B, or possibly Fluconazole, while cystitis may be successfully managed by bladder irrigation with amphotericin B or with oral fluconazole. Surgery may occasionally be necessary to remove obstructing fungus balls.

TABLE 4.2. DIAGNOSTIC CHART: BACTERIURIA AND PYURIA—SELECTED ETIOLOGIES

Disease	Epidemiology, Etiology, and/or Pathogenesis	Clinical Signs	Diagnosis	Initial Treatment (Alternative Rx in Parentheses)
A. Urethritis				
1. Gonococcal	Sexually transmitted to genitalia, rectum, or pharynx	Burning and difficulty on urination. Urethral discharge, usually purulent. Patient usually afebrile.	Males: Gram stain of urethral discharge. Gram-negative diplococci associated with PMNs. Positive culture is confirmatory, but not essential for diagnosis. Females: Positive culture from cervix or rectum required. PCR may prove useful.	Ceftriaxone IM Ciprofloxacin po (always follow gonococcal Rx with a course of doxycycline for the likely dual infection due to chlamydia).
2. Nonspecific (NSU)	Most are thought to be sexually transmitted. Chlamydia account for many of these infections.	Patient usually afebrile. Burning on urination. Urethral discharge, usually mucoid.	Combination of symptom-complex with negative smear and culture for gonococci and other pathogens such as Candida or Trichomonas, and no significant bacteriuria. Significant PMNs in urethral exudate or	Doxycycline po (erythromycin po)

BACTERIURIA AND PYURIA

3. Secondary to cystitis or pyelonephritis	Usually caused by Gram-negative aerobic rods.	Associated symptoms suggestive of UTI. initial voided urine. Chlamydia may be identified specifically by culture, antigen detection, nucleic acid hybridization & PCR, if available and cost-effective.	Same as treatment of UTI.
4. Candidal	Secondary to candidal cystitis or autoinfection from gut or vagina.	Burning on urination; urethral discharge. Gram stain of unspun urine (see text). Urine culture and colony count. Gram stain of discharge. KOH preparation of discharge; mix specimen with a drop of KOH and examine under microscope.	Insufficient data. Topical antifungal agents have been used in urethra and vagina. Role of po fluconazole not defined.
5. Trichomonal	Sexual transmission occurs.	Associated vaginitis in females and prostatitis in males. Patients usually afebrile, but complain of dysuria and urethral discharge. "Wet mount": mix urine, urethral and/or vaginal discharge with drop of saline and examine under microscope. Giemsa stain also helpful.	Flagyl (treat both partners simultaneously) (Avoid Flagyl in pregnancy)

(continued)

TABLE 4.2. *(continued)* DIAGNOSTIC CHART: BACTERIURIA AND PYURIA—SELECTED ETIOLOGIES

Disease	Epidemiology, Etiology, and/or Pathogenesis	Clinical Signs	Diagnosis	Initial Treatment (Alternative Rx in Parentheses)
B. Prostatitis (usually associated with seminal vesiculitis)				
1. Acute	Seen especially in young males. Usually spreads by direct extension from lower UTI (posterior urethritis). Infection may occur via the hematogenous route, especially with staphylococci. Predisposing factors include alcoholism, excessive sexual activity, or perineal trauma.	Fever, chills, dysuria and pain in rectum, back, perineum, and genitalia are common complaints. Prostate is tender, tense or boggy.	Culture urine and prostatic secretions. Avoid aggressive massage of acutely inflamed gland, but gentle pressure may produce a discharge for examination and culture done by a modified three-glass test may be helpful: after a midstream sterile collection of a urine specimen in which the bladder is emptied, prostatic massage is done, following which the patient's urine is again collected. Cells and bacteria in larger	Trimethoprim-sulfamethoxazole (unless antibiotic sensitivity testing dictates another choice). Sitz baths, fluids, and rest are indicated.

BACTERIURIA AND PYURIA

2. Chronic	Probably results from either repeated clinical or subclinical bouts of acute prostatitis. Is considered to be much less common than was previously thought.	Lumbar and perineal pain, dysuria, difficulty urinating with or without fever are common complaints. Prostate may be lightly tender and boggy on examination, but may be relatively normal.	Prostatic secretions contain many WBCs and bacteria. Urine and prostatic secretions have positive cultures. Modified three-glass test (described above) may be helpful. If tuberculosis is considered, culture of prostatic secretions is indicated, but acid-fast smear is not, because of the common presence of *Mycobacterium smegmatis*, a commensal in this area.	As above, with the exception that massage is thought to be helpful by some.
3. Non-bacterial prostatitis	No proven etiology.	Same as chronic prostatitis.	WBCs present in prostatic secretion, but no pathogens found, even on careful culture.	Doxycycline (erythromycin)

(continued)

Note: "numbers in specimen 2 than 1 are considered to be of prostatic origin." (continued from previous page)

TABLE 4.2. (continued) DIAGNOSTIC CHART: BACTERIURIA AND PYURIA—SELECTED ETIOLOGIES

Disease	Epidemiology, Etiology, and/or Pathogenesis	Clinical Signs	Diagnosis	Initial Treatment (Alternative Rx in Parentheses)
4. Prostatic abscess	Occurs secondary to acute prostatic infection.	Findings similar to acute prostatitis, but incomplete response to therapy or recrudescence of symptoms and signs. Urinary retention may occur. A fluctuant area may be felt in the prostate.	Blood, urine, and prostatic secretions should be cultured.	Surgical drainage via perineum (best) or transurethrally, and antibiotic therapy based on sensitivities. Trimethoprim-sulfamethoxazole is the drug of choice unless sensitivities dictate otherwise.
C. Symptomatic bacteriuria				
1. Cystitis	Primarily seen in females. Predisposing factors include obstruction, diabetes, instrumentation, catheterization, pregnancy, neurologic deficit, and sexual activity. Most common causes of infection are Gram-negative bacteria	Common symptoms include dysuria, frequency, nocturia, urgency, and pain in the perineal, suprapubic, or lumbar area. Suprapubic tenderness may be present. Urine can look cloudy and smell foul. Fever may be present,	Urine analysis with Gram stain of unspun sediment. Standard urine culture, colony counts, and sensitivity tests, (simplified bacteriologic and chemical tests are available for office use and are accurate and inexpenive for screening	Uncomplicated first infection: TMP-SMX, or tetracycline. Short course of therapy usually adequate (see text). Complicated infections: Treatment based on sensitivities. Parenteral antibiotics are indicated if bacteremia suspected.

or enterococci ascending the urethra from vaginal vestibule. Etiology: Uncomplicated first infection usually results from *E. coli.* Infections complicated by obstruction or instrumentation or recurrent episodes are also most commonly due to *E. coli,* but also result from Klebsiella, enterococcus, Proteus, Pseudomonas, and staphylococcus. The *E. coli* in these patients with complicated infection more likely show some increased antibiotic resistance over *E. coli* seen in uncomplicated UTI.

as may flank pain in some cases, and thus these findings do not necessarily indicate upper tract infection.

purposes). Women with recurrent infections, some children, and all males with UTI need urologic investigation. If bacteremia suspected blood cultures are indicated. Currently, simple laboratory tests are not available for differentiating upper vs. lower tract disease.

Force fluids for pyelonephritis. Establish adequate drainage if obstruction exists and correct lesion surgically if possible.

(continued)

TABLE 4.2. *(continued)* DIAGNOSTIC CHART: BACTERIURIA AND PYURIA—SELECTED ETIOLOGIES

Disease	Epidemiology, Etiology, and/or Pathogenesis	Clinical Signs	Diagnosis	Initial Treatment (Alternative Rx in Parentheses)
2. Pyelonephritis	Pathogenesis: usually ascending route from bladder, but may be secondary to bacteremia. Predisposing factors same as above, plus the following: renal trauma, medullary damage from hypokalemia, hypercalcemia, hypertension, diabetes, gout, acidosis, and certain drugs like phenacetin. Etiology: same as above.	Fever, chills, flank pain, dysuria; cloudy and foul-smelling urine; tenderness in flank and costovertebral areas are symptoms and signs suggestive of upper tract infection. All are not necessarily present, and some patients are asymptomatic. Furthermore, the presence of these symptoms may be found in some patients with only lower urinary tract disease.	Same as above.	Treat for 10 days to 2 weeks. If relapse occurs, longer course of therapy may be helpful (see text). May treat po if convenient drug available.
D. Papillary necrosis	Patients usually over 40 years old with one of the following associated diseases: infection, obstruction, diabetes	Usually chills, fever, flank pain, renal colic, abdominal pain, renal failure present, but symptoms may	Urinalysis: see WBCs, RBCs, bacteria. Strain urine and examine for tissue fragments. Imaging studies show	Antibiotics (ampicillin and gentamicin prior to report on sensitivities), supportive measures, correct obstruction.

	mellitus, interstitial nephritis, analgesic abuse, or sickle cell anemia.	sometimes be less dramatic. Passage of papillary fragments in the urine sometimes noted. Mortality rate is high because of uremia or septicemia.	deformed papillae, decreased excretory function, and enlarged renal silhouette. May see calcification representing previously infarcted papilla.	Occasionally partial or complete nephrectomy required.
E. Renal abscess				
1. Cortical	Usually results from staphylococcal bacteremia.	Chills, fever, flank pain and tenderness are classical. Another presentation is less dramatic with little or no symptomatology other than fever.	Urinalysis: Gram-positive cocci may be seen, with very few WBCs. Other useful procedures include blood cultures, sonograms, and CAT scan.	Vancomycin. May try intensive medical treatment first, but surgery needed in most cases.
2. Medullary	Results from pyelonephritis. Usually Gram-negative rods.	Chills, fever, costovertebral angle pain and tenderness.	Urinalysis: Gram-negative bacilli seen, with numerous WBCs; other tests found useful include blood cultures, sonogram, CAT scan.	Gentamicin and ampicillin prior to report on cultures and sensitivities.

(continued)

TABLE 4.2. (continued) DIAGNOSTIC CHART: BACTERIURIA AND PYURIA—SELECTED ETIOLOGIES

Disease	Epidemiology, Etiology, and/or Pathogenesis	Clinical Signs	Diagnosis	Initial Treatment (Alternative Rx in Parentheses)
F. Perinephric abscess	Two-thirds result from extension of pyelonephritis; one-third results from hematogenous spread, usually with staphylococci. Associated with diabetes, renal calculi.	Insidious illness with fever, flank pain, dysuria, flank mass, or tenderness. Should be suspected after prolonged course of "pyelonephritis" that is unresponsive to appropriate antimicrobial therapy.	Urinalysis shows abnormalities in only 75%. Blood cultures positive in 40%. Urine cultures positive in 70% KUB of abdomen abnormal in 50%—see mass or absent psoas shadow. Chest x-ray is abnormal in 50%—see pleural effusion, lower lobe infiltrate, elevated diaphragm on the affected side. Sonogram or CT scan helpful.	Surgical drainage. Antibiotics, choice depending on culture results or suspected pathogens, if culture results not available. If associated with *S. aureus* bacteremia, vancomycin. If associated with Gram-negative rod pyelonephritis, gentamicin, tobramycin, or amikacin is chosen until sensitivities available.
G. Candida Infections				
1. Cystitis	Associated with indwelling catheters, prior antibiotic therapy, and corticosteroid administration. Usually secondary to urethral	Dyuria, frequency, nocturia, cloudy urine, urgency, and pain in perineal, suprapubic or lumbar areas are presenting findings if	Culture: catheterized urine or suprapubic bladder aspirate most reliable. Colony count of modest help.	Usually presence of Candida in urine requires no specific therapy. Frequently clears on its own after antibiotics are

	contamination by vaginal or fecal flora.	symptomatic, but usually infection is asymptomatic.	discontinued and the catheter removed. If candiduria is symptomatic or persistent or if cystocopy shows marked involvement of bladder wall, bladder irrigation with amphotericin B or systemic treatment with fluconazole may be used.
2. Pyelonephritis	Usually ascending, but may be hematogenous. Associated with indwelling catheters, antibiotics, corticosteroid administration, prior GU surgery, underlying renal disease.	Fever and chills may be present with flank pain, dysuria, cloudy urine, and tender CVA. Search for evidence of possible disseminated candidiasis should include ophthalmoscopic exam for typical retinal lesions, careful search for skin lesions, and repeat blood cultures.	Urine culture of catherized specimen or suprapubic bladder aspirate is most reliable. Colony count of modest help. Blood cultures indicated. Sonogram or CT scan may be abnormal, demonstrating characteristic fungus balls. Serology may help in diagnosis of disseminated disease.	Stop antibiotics and remove catheters and foreign bodies if possible. Amphotericin B is drug of choice. Fluconazole may be substituted if organism is sensitive. Surgery may be required to remove fungus balls.

(continued)

TABLE 4.2. (continued) DIAGNOSTIC CHART: BACTERIURIA AND PYURIA—SELECTED ETIOLOGIES

Disease	Epidemiology, Etiology, and/or Pathogenesis	Clinical Signs	Diagnosis	Initial Treatment (Alternative Rx in Parentheses)
H. GU tuberculosis	Kidney involvement frequently results from hematogenous spread at the time of initial pulmonary infection, but GU tract infection might not manifest itself for many years. Organisms then spread from upper urinary tract to the lower tract via the urine.	Most frequently, patients have the symptoms of cystitis or pyelonephritis described above. Some patients have primarily pulmonary symptoms or may be totally asymptomatic.	Suspect with "sterile" pyuria. Hematuria frequently present. Urine culture negative for usual bacterial pathogens in most, but positive for TB in 80%. Sputum culture positive in 40%. Pulmonary disease evident in 50%. Skin test is positive in majority of cases. Cystoscopy may prove bladder involvement if ulcerations and submucosal tubercles are seen. IVP is abnormal in most cases and in some is highly characteristic.	Isoniazid, rifampin, pyrazinamide and ethambutol. Surgery may be necessary for (a) relief of obstruction and/or (b) poor response to medical therapy. Hypertension may rarely be attributed to tuberculous kidney disease, and after careful study surgery may prove efficacious in some patients.

5

DIARRHEA

Diarrhea may be defined as the passage of poorly formed stools, a disorder ranging from a trivial inconvenience to an acute, life-threatening emergency. Infectious diarrheal diseases are frequently caused by viruses or bacterial infections and may be divided conveniently into three groups: noninflammatory, inflammatory, and penetrating (Table 5.1).

GENERAL FEATURES
Noninflammatory Diarrhea

This type of diarrhea is caused by toxin-producing bacteria, viruses, and some parasites. Disease is limited to the small bowel, where the absorptive capability of the villi is impaired, with an outpouring of fluid and electrolytes. No mucosal invasion occurs, and minimal, if any, histologic changes are seen on small bowel biopsy. Systemic symptoms such as fever, malaise and anorexia are mild or absent. Periumbilical pain, profuse watery stools and gaseous distension are manifestations of small bowel involvement.

Inflammatory Diarrhea

On the other hand, the invasive pathogens (e.g., Shigella, invasive *E. coli*) actually infect and destroy the mucosa, especially of the

DIFFERENTIAL DIAGNOSIS OF INFECTIOUS DISEASES

TABLE 5.1. TYPE OF ENTERIC INFECTION

	Non-inflammatory	Inflammatory	Penetrating
Site	Small bowel	Colon	Ileum (lymphoid tissue)
WBCs	No	PMNs	Mononuclear cells
Syndrome	Large volume diarrhea	Dysentery	Enteric fever
EXAMPLES	E. coli (toxigenic) V. cholerae Rotavirus Norwalk-like virus Giardia Staph food poisoning Clostridium food poisoning Cryptosporidium & related protozoa Heavy metals Mushroom poisoning Fish & shellfish poisoning	Shigella Salmonella C. Jejuni E. coli (invasive) C. difficile toxin Amebiasis	S. typhi Yersinia C. fetus

colon. Therefore, initial watery diarrhea and other mild symptoms related to small bowel involvement may be followed by colonic symptoms such as cramps, tenesmus, rectal urgency, and the passage of mucoid stools, at times with blood. Fever and constitutional signs are usually more prominent in this condition than in toxin-induced disease.

Penetrating Diarrhea

A third type of diarrhea results from bacteria that penetrate the intestinal mucosa (usually in the ileum) but do not destroy it.

Enteric fever, a systemic infection of which typhoid fever is the prototype, results from this distinctive pathophysiology.

Fecal Leukocytes

The differences in pathophysiology described above are important, for they explain the differences found on examination of the stool. Damage to the mucosa (e.g., from bacteria that cause inflammatory diarrhea), causes an outpouring of polymorphonuclear leukocytes which may be seen on Wright's stain of a fresh stool specimen. Methylene blue stain is particularly useful in this setting, and newly-developed techniques such as stool testing for lactoferrin may facilitate the detection of polymorphs. In contrast to this, illnesses resulting from viruses or enterotoxigenic bacteria produce no or few WBCs in the feces. In penetrating bacterial disease, the WBCs that are shed in the stool are predominantly lymphocytes.

Host Factors

The factors thought to predispose a patient to microbial invasion of the intestinal tract are many, including subnormal gastric acidity, poor intestinal motility, derangement of normal intestinal flora, and deficient coproantibodies.

Before considering specific causes of diarrhea, it is important to remember that diarrhea may at times be a nonspecific response to a severe infection elsewhere in the body. This nonspecific diarrheal response to infection is most frequently seen in infants, but may occur in adults, especially with Gram-negative sepsis or severe pyelonephritis.

KNOWN CAUSES OF DIARRHEAL DISEASES
(Table 5.2)

Noninflammatory

Most infectious diarrhea in the United States is noninflammatory, resulting from toxins or viral infection. Fortunately, illnesses

TABLE 5.2. DIARRHEA

1. Non-inflammatory (small bowel)
   a. Viruses
      1. Rotoviruses
      2. Parvoviruses (Norwalk)
   b. Toxigenic bacteria
      1. S. aureus
      2. C. perfringens
      3. V. cholerae
      4. E. Coli
      5. B. cereus
   c. Parasites
      1. Giardia and others (Ascaris, hookworm, Strongyloides, Taenia, Trichinella, Cryptosporidia, etc.)

2. Inflammatory (large bowel)
   a. Bacteria
      1. Shigella
      2. E. Coli
      3. Salmonella
      4. Yersinia
      5. Campylobacter
      6. S. aureus
      7. V. parahaemoliticus
      8. C. difficile
   b. Parasites
      1. E. histolytica and others (*Balantidium coli,* schistosoma)

3. Enteric fever
   a. *Salmonella typhi*
   b. *Campylobacter jejuni*
   c. Yersinia enterocolitica

caused by these agents are usually mild and self-limited, although they may be devastating in young children and infants.

Viral Gastroenteritis

Viruses are leading causes of infectious diarrhea, especially in young children during the winter months. The major viral groups involved are the rotaviruses (the reovirus, orbivirus) and parvoviruses. The rotaviruses usually cause a short-term acute illness with mild nausea, vomiting, and prominent diarrhea. The illness may be accompanied by fever and cramps. The parvoviruses have been implicated as the cause of several outbreaks of "winter vomiting disease." Adenoviruses and enteroviruses have also been reported to produce diarrhea on rare occasions. Fecal leukocytes are uncommonly associated with viral gastroenteritis.

Staphylococcal Food Poisoning

Staphylococcal food poisoning occurs a few hours after ingesting preformed staphylococcal toxins, usually in contaminated meat or cream-containing food. A relatively mild illness lasting 6 to 24 hours results. Nausea, vomiting, and saline depletion are more prominent than the diarrhea. Significant fever is rare.

Clostridial Diarrhea

C. perfringens causes a mild gastroenteritis with marked diarrhea but little nausea and vomiting. The ingested organisms form the toxin *in vivo*, producing symptoms in about 12 hours. This diagnosis should be suspected especially after eating reheated meat and poultry dishes. The usual hospital laboratory is rarely set up to test for enterotoxin-producing clostridia.

Cholera

Cholera is seen in many areas of the world, where it may be present in epidemic proportions. In the United States, it is seen occasionally in southern states, e.g., Louisiana and Texas. It is generally associated with deficient sanitation and is manifested by severe watery diarrhea. Significant fever is lacking, but the profuse diarrhea (liters) can be fatal in hours. Vigorous fluid and electrolyte repletion can reduce mortality to 1 percent or less. Cholera is caused by an enterotoxin produced *in vivo* by *V. cholerae*. Fecal leukocytes are not seen with this noninvasive infection.

E. Coli

Enterotoxigenic *E. coli* (ETEC) produce a heat-labile and a heat-stable toxin. They are the most common bacterial cause of acute diarrhea in the world, and are respnsible for most cases of traveler's diarrhea, or "turista." The disease begins after an incubation period of 8 to 44 hours and is manifested by voluminous watery diarrhea for 12 to 72 hours. Enterohemorrhagic *E. coli* (EHEC) causes a noninflammatory diarrhea (no fever, no stool WBCs) but it is a serious disorder in that the diarrhea may become grossly hemorrhagic, and the hemolytic-uremic syndrome or TTP may develop, with appreciable mortality. Outbreaks have occurred attributed to undercooked meat. Serotype 0157:H7 is the most common, but not the only identified serotype. The organism's ferocity is attributed to production of Shiga-like toxins. *E. coli* also causes a noninflammatory diarrhea by several types of adherence, i.e., local (EPEC strains), aggregative (EAggEC strains), or diffuse (DAEC) adherence to intestinal mucosa.

Bacillus cereus

B. cereus also causes a toxogenic diarrhea, often associated with fried rice and other grains. It produces illness of both short and long incubation periods, the latter typically associated with prominent diarrhea.

The toxigenic bacteria discussed above (*E. coli, C. perfringens, S. aureus, B. cereus* and *V. cholerae*) do not cause invasive disease, and therefore, examination of the stools of these patients will not usually show fecal leukocytes.

Specific Inflammatory Diarrheas

Inflammatory bacterial diarrheas are less common, but are more likely to be diagnosed because of readily available laboratory methodology. This group includes invasive *E. coli* diarrhea, shigellosis, salmonellosis, staphylococcal enterocolitis, and antimicrobial-induced pseudomembranous colitis caused by *Clostridium difficile*.

Invasive Infections: Shigellosis and Certain *E. Coli*

Shigella is the classical prototype of an organism causing "dysentery" or a "dysentery-like" illness. This bacterium is usually spread by person-to-person contact in areas of poor sanitation or by food and water contaminated by human carriers. Shigellae typically produce the abrupt onset of headache, cramps, fever, mucoid diarrhea that may be bloody, tenesmus, and at times, mild nausea and vomiting. This illness results primarily from the direct invasion of the colonic mucosa, although some toxin production probably contributes to the overall toxicity. Diffuse mucosal ulceration and hemorrhage may be seen on sigmoidoscopy.

Some strains of *E. coli* (Enteroinvasive *E. coli* or EIEC) can directly infect the GI tract and produce a disease indistinguishable from shigellosis. Such invasive strains of *E. coli* may be detected in several simple animal tests, but are not tested for routinely in most hospital laboratories.

Salmonellosis

Salmonella gastroenteritis is caused by salmonellae other than *S. typhi* and is characterized by fever, diarrhea, and cramps usually occurring within 24 hours after ingestion of the agent. In salmonella gastroenteritis the stools rarely contain blood and mucous. This disease is almost always mild and self limited, but on occasion may cause a severe, ulcerative colitis-like illness. The disease may be especially severe in the very old or young or those with other underlying illnesses, particularly malignancy, or with defective immune status, for example AIDS. Rarely, salmonella gastroenteritis may produce an appendicitis-like picture. Unlike *S. typhi*, which is found only in man, the other salmonellae are widespread in nature, and infection in man is frequently related to ingestion of contaminated animal products.

Yersinia enterocolitica Infection

Yersinia enterocolitica may produce a severe febrile diarrheal syndrome which at times may be mistaken for appendicitis because of the acute mesenteric adenitis which may involve the terminal ileum. Many patients have had appendectomies because of this confusing syndrome. Diarrhea is rarely bloody, but frequently contains PMLs. At times the disease has been thought to be related to pathogens from animals such as dogs, or to contaminated foods such as chocolate milk. In certain patients, arthritis and/or rashes such as erythema nodosum may occur with or without the diarrhea. Special studies are required to detect the organism in the stool and antibiotic susceptibility studies are always indicated since sensitivities are quite variable.

Campylobacter jejuni

Campylobacter jejuni is a relatively common bacterial cause of inflammatory enteritis. The diarrhea may be bloody and thus suggest idiopathic ulcerative colitis. Severe pain in the right lower quadrant of the abdomen may suggest Crohn's disease or appendicitis, especially when present in young patients.

Staphylococcal Enterocolitis

In patients rendered susceptible by surgery, shock, or prior antibiotics, *S. aureus* may multiply in the GI tract and produce a severe colitis. When this diagnosis is suspected, Gram staining of the stool must be done to look for the large numbers of PMLs and clumps of Gram-positive cocci. Those factors predisposing to intestinal invasion by the staphylococcus occasionally may allow a similar invasion and severe colitis by other colonic flora, especially proteus, pseudomonas, and *C. albicans*.

Vibrio parahaemolyticus

Vibrio parahaemolyticus may also cause an invasive diarrhea, typically associated with ingestion of contaminated shellfish. Toxins may also play a role in this illness, characterized by fever, diarrhea, abdominal cramps, and vomiting.

The diseases just discussed all produce their symptoms by direct invasion of the intestinal mucosa. Therefore, examination of the stool in patients with disease caused by Shigella, Salmonella, invasive *E. coli*, Yersinia, Campylobacter, and colitis-producing staphylococci may show leukocytes. The WBCs will be polymorphonuclear in all cases except those caused by *S. typhi*, in which case mononuclear cells are seen.

On occasion a toxin-induced syndrome may produce severe colitis which may mimic the invasive disorders discussed above. Thus, the pseudomembranous colitis caused by *C. difficile* may produce fever and stool leukocytes; this entity is discussed below under antibiotic-induced diarrhea.

The entity of infectious proctitis can mimic inflammatory enterocolitis. This should be suspected particularly in male homosexuals who engage in rectal intercourse. Gonorrhea, syphilis, chlamydial and herpetic infection can all be spread via this behavior and can cause severe proctitis.

The most important noninfectious disease that must be considered in the differential diagnosis of severe diarrheal disease with WBCs in the stool is idiopathic ulcerative colitis. The sigmoidoscopic appearance may not distinguish this entity from a shigella-like illness.

Penetrating (enteric fever)

The enteric fevers are represented by *S. typhi*, though other Salmonella serotypes can be etiologic. Typically, after a 1- to 2-week incubation period, patients develop headache, fever and cramps. Although diarrhea occurs, many patients present with constipation. Other "clues" to typhoid fever are rose spots (truncal red papules that blanch with pressure), hepatosplenomegaly, leukopenia, relative bradycardia and rarely, cough and epistaxis.

On occasion, Yersinia and *C. jejuni* may produce enteric fever, as may *Pseudomonas aeruginosa* ("Shanghai Fever").

As noted, some of the causes of invasive diarrhea and enteric fever can produce mesenteric adenitis and a resultant *pseudoappendicitis*. CT scan may sometimes be helpful, in addition to stool and blood cultures. Major causes of this presentation are salmonella, *Campylobacter jejuni* and Yersinia. Extreme abdominal pain associated with bloody or watery diarrhea may also represent the entity of *typhlitis*, inflammation of the cecum in patients with neutropenia.

PARASITIC CAUSES OF GASTROENTERITIS

A number of parasites can cause diarrheal disease, and a careful examination of the patient's stool (not rectal swab) is essential. If one is looking for motile trophozoites, it is best to examine a drop of warm fresh feces diluted in saline; if the procedure cannot be done immediately, the specimen should be preserved in a fixative (polyvinyl alcohol) either on a slide or in a bottle. In this manner, the trophozoites may remain visible, although their characteristic motility will be lost. Trophozoites are more likely to be found if diarrhea is present.

A wet mount prepared with a drop of dilute iodine solution is helpful in the study of cyst forms. If formed stools are passed, cysts are far more likely to be seen than trophozoites. Temporary refrigeration of a formed stool is acceptable, as the cysts will remain intact. Cysts are most effectively demonstrated by concentration with a formalin-ether mixture. This mixture destroys trophozoites, but should be used when examining a formed stool for cysts. It is also helpful in examining a stool specimen for the eggs of helminths or for larvae (especially important in strongyloidiasis).

Nuclear stains, such as iron hematoxylin or trichrome stain, are important to determine the taxonomic features of cysts and trophozoites. Modified acid fast stains are used to detect Cryptosporidium, Isopora, mycobacteria and Cyanobacteria, pathogens important in AIDS patients with diarrhea. However, Cryptosporidium and Cyanobacteria (formerly referred to as blue-green algae) are also seen in immunocompetent individuals, in whom they may cause a self limited noninflammatory diarrhea.

It is important to note that repeated specimens (usually at least three to six) are necessary to evaluate a stool for parasites, but the absence of parasites, even on numerous stool examinations, does not necessarily rule out the possibility of parasitic infection. Two parasites, Giardia and Strongyloides, occasionally require examination of duodenal fluid or biopsy to establish the diagnosis.

Of the many parasitic causes of diarrhea, there are two protozoal diseases that are reviewed here because of their relative frequency in the United States and their potential severity: amebiasis and giardiasis. (A group of protozoal diarrheas that are a particular problem in AIDS—cryptosporidium, isospora, cyclospora and microsporidia—may on occasion cause disease in immunocompetent hosts; one of these, cyclospora, is emerging as a cause of traveler's diarrhea.)

Amebiasis

E. histolytica usually causes a chronic diarrhea, but may produce an illness that can be acute, with fever, diarrhea, and bloody stools. In the United States it must be considered especially in patients who live in poor sanitary conditions or who have traveled to Mexico, Central America, Africa, Asia, or the Middle East. A fresh stool should be examined as described above. Sigmoidoscopic findings are sometimes characteristic and careful examination of mucous from an ulcer crater may reveal motile trophozoites. Mucosal biopsy may be necessary to demonstrate the organism. In invasive bowel infection, the indirect hemagglutination test performed on the patient's serum is positive in most cases, but should not substitute for demonstration of the organism.

Giardiasis

Giardia lamblia is capable of producing infections ranging from asymptomatic colonization to chronic diarrheal disease with nausea, malabsorption, and weight loss. The infection is superficial and noninflammatory. Giardiasis may be seen in epidemic form and should be suspected particularly in patients who have been drinking from freshwater streams. Person-to-person spread in situations such as nursery schools has also been reported. A smear of the stool will usually demonstrate the parasite, but sometimes duodenal mucosal biopsy or aspirate is needed to make the diagnosis.

Many other parasites may produce diarrheal illness. Patients who have traveled to or lived in endemic areas and/or who demonstrate eosinophilia should raise suspicion of a helminthic infestation, and stool examination for the organism or its eggs should be undertaken.

Although associated more with abdominal pain and vomiting than with diarrhea, the entity of infective gastritis is another form of gastrointestinal infection and results from direct invasion of the gastric mucosa. The organisms most commonly responsible are *Helicobacter pylori* (a treatable cause of duodenal ulcer, gastric ulcer, and gastritis), *T. pallidum* (especially during the course of secondary syphilis), *M. tuberculosis* and, in AIDS patients, cytomegalovirus.

Antibiotic-Induced Diarrhea

Occasionally a patient receiving antibiotic therapy will develop diarrhea as a complication of treatment. A small proportion of these patients will have diarrhea caused by a toxin produced by *C. difficile*. Rarely, the toxin causes more severe disease in the form of ileus, megacolon or colitis with characteristic pseudomembranes seen on endoscopy. Discontinuation of the offending antibiotic (usually ampicillin, clindamycin or cephalosporins, but others can do it) usually suffices, but some patients require therapy with oral vancomycin or metronidazole. *C. difficile*-related diarrhea may cause WBCs in the stool. Further, it may occur in patients who have not received antibiotics but who are susceptible because they are post-operative, have underlying malignancy, etc. Anti-motility agents should be avoided.

TOXIN-INDUCED GASTROENTERITIS

Several toxins may cause gastroenteritis when ingested and must be considered in the differential diagnosis of acute diarrhea with minimal constitutional signs: (a) heavy metals (see chart) may produce nausea, vomiting, and diarrhea minutes to hours after ingestion; (b) mushroom poisoning results in a gastroenteritis accompanied by the muscarinic symptoms of salivation, sweating, miosis, and bradycardia in 6 to 12 hours; (c) fish poisoning can produce nausea, vomiting and diarrhea in hours, accompanied by numbness and pruritus in the ciguatera type and by a histamine-like reaction in the scombroid variety; (d) when a neurologic syndrome that is predominantly motor follows acute nausea, vomiting and diarrhea, botulism should always be considered. Table 5.3 lists these and other noninfectious causes of diarrhea.

Non-specific Therapy

Non-specific therapy for diarrhea should include avoidance of anti-diarrheal medication if possible, and repletion of fluid and electrolyte loss. An oral formulation that contains glucose, sodium chloride, bicarbonate, and potassium or a cereal-based solution that replaces the glucose with rice or wheat or mashed boiled potatoes has been found useful in rehydrating, reversing fluid loss and preventing hypoglycemia in children. The basic solution can be approximated by the combination of 1 tsp table salt, 1 tsp of baking soda, 1 cup of orange juice, and 4 tbsp of sugar, all added to 1 quart (liter) of water.

TABLE 5.3. NONINFECTIOUS CAUSES OF DIARRHEA

A. Drugs
   1. Antibiotics
   2. Cathartics
   3. Cholinergics
   4. Thyroid replacement
   5. Antimetabolites

B. Irritating Foods

C. Poisoning
   1. Fish
   2. Mushrooms
   3. Heavy metals

D. Miscellaneous
   1. Functional bowel disturbances
   2. Ulcerative colitis
   3. Ischemic colitis
   4. Pellagra
   5. Lower GI hemorrhage
   6. Disaccharidase deficiencies (may be postinfectious)
   7. Henoch-Schonlein purpura
   8. Hyperthyroidism
   9. Adrenal insufficiency
   10. Allergy
   11. Necrotizing enterocolitis

TABLE 5.4. DIAGNOSTIC CHART: DIARRHEA—SELECTED ETIOLOGIES

Disease or Organism	Pathogenesis	Epidemiology	Clinical Signs	Diagnosis	Initial Therapy (Alternate Rx in Parentheses)
A. Viral gastroenteritis	Non-inflammatory	Person-to-person spread. Perhaps most important cause of diarrhea in young children, especially during the winter months. May cause epidemics of disease and may spread in the hospital. Some cases due to parvovirus present with severe vomiting.	16–48 hour incubation; causes variable degrees of fever, diarrhea, vomiting, and cramps. Bloody stools uncommon.	No fecal leukocytes. Diagnosis can be made by electron or immune electron microscopy. Serologic methods being developed.	Supportive therapy.
B. *E. coli* diarrhea	Enterotoxigenic (ETEC). Activation of cyclic AMP with increased secretion of fluid and electrolytes into gut lumen. Non-inflammatory.	Food and water, human source.	24–72 hour incubation, watery diarrhea, and minimal fever, important cause of "turista" or traveler's diarrhea.	No fecal leukocytes; not specifically diagnosable in most clinical laboratories. Serotyping of *E. coli* of uncertain value clinically, but clearly of epidemiologic significance.	Symptomatic. Pepto-Bismol, quinolones.
	Enteroinvasive (EIEC). Inflammatory destruction of large bowel mucosa.	Person-to-person, food and water. Some outbreaks in U.S. related to cheeses.	24–72 hour incubation, fever, mucoid and at times bloody diarrhea, tenesmus.	Abundant fecal leukocytes (PMNS); positive screening test conjunctivitis in guinea pigs. Not specifically diagnosable in most clinical labs. Serotyping of uncertain value clinically but may be of epidemiologic importance.	Symptomatic. In severe cases, quinolones, TMP-SMX.

DIARRHEA

	Enterohemmorrhagic (EHEC).	Food-borne.	Bloody diarrhea. No fever. Occasional hemolytic-uremic syndrome. TTP.	No fecal WBCs. Suspect in outbreaks. Serotype 0157:H7.	Quinolones. TMP-SMX (efficiency not proven).
C. *S. aureus* food poisoning	Enterotoxin production. Non-inflammatory.	Foods contaminated by food handler with staphylococcal infection.	2–6 hour incubation; vomiting and cramps with minimal diarrhea.	Clinical diagnosis. Food may be studied for presence of enterotoxin-producing staphylococci, as may be stool of infected patients.	Symptomatic therapy.
D. Cholera	Toxigenic: Activation of cyclic AMP, with increased secretion of fluid and electrolytes into gut lumen.	Contaminated food and water from human source. Most cases occur in the Indian subcontinent, the Far East, and Middle East. Some spread into the African continent. Occasional cases seen in Europe and the U.S.	24–48 hour incubation. Afebrile; severe fluid and electrolyte loss due to massive watery diarrhea.	No fecal leukocytes. Organism grown from stool or rectal swabs on special agar. May diagnose with direct fluorescent antibody studies on stool specimens.	Massive fluid and electrolyte support. Doxycycline (TMP-SMX, quinolones).
E. *C. perfringens* diarrhea	Enterotoxin-producing strains. Non-inflammatory.	Food-borne. Contaminated foods, especially warmed-over meats.	4–24 hour incubation, afebrile, and watery, self-limited diarrhea.	No fecal leukocytes. Organism isolated from stool and evaluated for presence of toxin formation. Not specifically diagnosable by most clinical laboratories.	Symptomatic therapy.

(continued)

TABLE 5.4. (continued) DIAGNOSTIC CHART: DIARRHEA—SELECTED ETIOLOGIES

Disease or Organism	Pathogenesis	Epidemiology	Clinical Signs	Diagnosis	Initial Therapy (Alternate Rx in Parentheses)
F. *B. cereus* diarrhea	Toxigenic. (Perhaps two toxins: one of short and one of long duration).	Fried rice implicated in short-incubation-disease. Other grains implicated in long-incubation disease.	Afebrile. Two types of syndromes noted: (1) short incubation, 3-6 hours, with nausea and vomiting; (2) a longer incubation, 12-24 hours, with diarrhea as a prominent feature.	Case usually proven only in epidemic settings. Organism must be demonstrated in high titre ($>10^5$) in food.	Supportive.
G. Giardiasis	Marked proliferation of organism in upper small bowel producing malabsorption. Non-inflammatory.	Human: person-to-person spread and waterborne outbreaks reported (especially in travelers from the former U.S.S.R.).	1-3 week incubation. Symptoms vary from none to midepigastric pain, flatulence, anorexia, severe malabsorption, and weight loss.	Organism seen in stool in many cases. If negative, need do duodenal aspirate and biopsies with special stains and preparations. No serology available.	Quinacrine. (metronidazole.)
H. Cryptosporidia and related protozoa, e.g., isospora, cyclospora, and microsporidia.	Small bowel-mucosal involvement.	Cryptosporidia associated with swimming in lakes, streams, and swimming pools (resistant to chlorine). Cyclospora emerging as a cause of traveler's diarrhea.	Chronic diarrhea. Cryptosporidia may also involve hepatobiliary tract, and microsporidia can involve liver, bile ducts, muscle & eye.	Stool smears for AFB for cryptosporidia, isospora & cyclospora. Small bowel biopsy may be required. Microsporidia is demonstrated by gram stain of stool or biopsy (resembles gram-positive neisseria).	Crypto: paromomycin Isospora: TMP-SMX Cyclospora: ?TMP-SMX Microsporidium: Albendazole, metronidazole.

DIARRHEA 129

I. Shigellosis	Inflammatory	Human (occasionally other primates). Person-to-person spread or food and water from a human source.	24–72 hour incubation. Fever; mucoid and at times bloody diarrhea; tenesmus.	Abundant fecal leukocytes (PMLs); positive stool or rectal swab culture. Rectal swabs better than stool for culture of shigellae. May use direct fluorescent antibody on stool to look for shigellae.	Check sensitivities, since these vary greatly from place to place and strain to strain. Quinolones, TMP-SMX.
J. Salmonellosis (nontyphoidal)	Inflammatory	Nonhuman animal sources (especially poultry, eggs, turtles, contaminated grain). Usually spread via contaminated food.	12–24 hour incubation. Mild fever, loose diarrhea, some cramping. Can see pseudo appendicitis, and, rarely, ulcerative colitis-like picture.	Fecal leukocytes somewhat increased (mostly PMLs). Stool or rectal swab cultures.	No antibiotics unless patient is very ill.
K. *Y. enterocolitica*	Primarily invasive, with lymphatic involvement, especially of the mesenteric nodes.	Contaminated water and food such as milk. Largest outbreak in US related to chocolate milk. May be related to animal contact as well.	Syndrome of fever, diarrhea; right lower quadrant pain simulating appendicitis especially suggestive. At times may be associated with skin rashes, including erythema nodosum. Can cause "enteric fever".	Fecal leukocytes usually present. Must notify lab so special cultures of stool with cold incubation can be done. Blood cultures may be helpful.	Supportive therapy. Antibiotics may be useful, but sensitivities quite variable. Aminoglycosides like gentamicin are effective against most strains.

(continued)

130 DIFFERENTIAL DIAGNOSIS OF INFECTIOUS DISEASES

TABLE 5.4. (continued) DIAGNOSTIC CHART: DIARRHEA–SELECTED ETIOLOGIES

Disease or Organism	Pathogenesis	Epidemiology	Clinical Signs	Diagnosis	Initial Therapy (Alternate Rx in Parentheses)
L. *C. jejuni*	Invasion of mucosa. Inflammatory. Involves both the large and small bowel.	Related to animals, foods.	Diarrhea, abdominal pain, fever, stools may be bloody. Can see mesenteric adenitis or enteric fever syndrome, also.	Stool culture.	Not needed in all patients. If Rx use erythromycin (quinolones).
M. *S. aureus* enterocolitis	Inflammatory	Patient usually receiving antibiotic resulting in overgrowth of *S. aureus*.	Ulcerative colitis picture with severe diarrhea. May develop shock or toxic megacolon.	Fecal leukocytes and sheets of staphylococci on Gram stain.	Stop prior antibiotics; begin oral vancomycin and parenteral anti-staphylococcal penicillin and appropriate fluid replacement.
N. *V. parahemolyticus*	Mucosal invasion with destruction. Toxins may play a role.	Contaminated shellfish.	10–20 hour incubation. Fever, diarrhea, vomiting and cramps are all common findings.	Fecal leukocytes present in some cases. Must notify lab for special cultures to be done.	Supportive.
O. *C. difficile*	Toxin produced by *C. difficile*.	Seen in patients receiving antibiotics; especially ampicillin, cephalosporins and	Abdominal pain, fever, diarrhea, rarely megacolon.	Toxin assay available. Fecal leukocytes present ½ the time.	Oral vancomycin (metronidazole), remove offending drug if possible.

DIARRHEA

P. Amebiasis	Invasive: large bowel.	Human contamination of food or water. Not usually cause of large epidemics.	Symptoms vary from no to marked fever, from constipation to mucoid or bloody diarrhea.	Trophozoites seen on smear (wet prep or special stain of stool or lesions swabbed at sigmoidoscopy or from biopsies). Serology helpful in invasive disease.	Metronidazole followed by diiodohydroxyquin.
Q. Typhoid fever (S. typhi)	Penetrating: Inflammation of lamina propria and bacteremia.	Human source. In the U.S., spread usually via food or water contamination by an elderly chronic S. typhi carrier.	10–14 day incubation. Fever; constipation or mild diarrhea; abdominal pain, splenomegaly, leukopenia with relative lymphocytosis. Pulse-temperature dissociation may occur. Rose spots, bowel perforations, hemorrhage, and metastatic infections may occur.	Blood, bone marrow, stool cultures; cultures on special media; fecal mononuclear cells are increased.	Depending on sensitivities, may be TMP-SMX, ciprofloxacin, or ceftriaxone. Some still prefer chloramphenicol.

(Row above P: ...clindamycin. Also seen post-op and in patients on cancer chemotherapy.)

6

RASH

The presence of a rash in an acutely ill febrile patient demands consideration of a wide spectrum of infectious diseases, ranging from a self limited benign infection caused by an enterovirus to a rapidly fatal infection such as meningococcemia. Most rashes encountered in the course of infectious illnesses are associated with viral diseases that require no specific treatment. On the other hand, there are some extremely serious diseases that cause rashes and require specific antimicrobial therapy. The emphasis in this chapter is on the latter group of diseases. Localized skin infections, e.g., cellulitis and ulcerating lesions are furnished in tabular form, but the emphasis is on diffuse eruptions, i.e., rashes. Furthermore, only those illnesses likely to be encountered in the United States are stressed.

For the purpose of this discussion, diseases are categorized by the type of rash produced (Table 6.1). The first group of rashes to be discussed are those of the petechial, purpuric or purpuric-vesicular type.

PETECHIAL AND PURPURIC RASHES

When seen in the acutely ill febrile patient, these skin findings should alert the physician to the possibility of an extremely serious disease.

TABLE 6.1. RASH

Petechiae/Purpura/Purpuric Vesicles[a]	Macules/Papules[b]	Vesicles/Bullae/Pustules[c]	Diffuse Erythema	Urticaria
		Specific Treatment Available		
Bacteremia (with or without DIC) Infectious endocarditis	Typhoid fever	Staphylococcemia	Streptococcal infection	Mycoplasma
Meningococcemia				
Gonococcemia	Secondary syphilis	Gonococcemia	Staphylococcal infection	Lyme disease
Other pathogenic bacteria	Early MnG	Rickettsialpox		
RMSF	Mycoplasma	Varicella-zoster	Ehrlichiosis	
Epidemic typhus	Lyme disease	Herpes simplex	S. viridans	
Rat-bite fevers	Rickettsiosis	Vibrio vulnificus	A. hemolyticum	
	Early RMSF			
	Epidemic typhus		Kawasaki disease	
	Brill-Zinsser disease			
	Murine typhus			
	R. Conorii			
	Ehrlichiosis			

No Specific Treatment Available

Enteroviral infection	Enteroviral infection	Enteroviral infection	Enteroviral infection	Enteroviral infection
Dengue	Parvovirus B19 (fifth disease)	Parvovirus B19		Adenovirus
Hepatitis	HHV-6	HIV		EBV
Rubella	Rubeola			HIV
EBV	Rubella			Hepatitis
	Adenovirus			
	EBV			
	HIV (Primary)			

[a] Diseases rarely causing these lesions: Murine typhus, psittacosis, tularemia, plague, congenital syphilis, malaria, disseminated histoplasmosis, miliary TB, brucellosis, leptospiriosis, *Vibrio vulnificus*, *R. conorii*.
[b] Diseases rarely causing these lesions: psittacosis, trichinosis, acquired toxoplasmosis, leptospirosis, leprosy
[c] Diseases rarely causing these lesions: *R. conorii*

The red or purple pigmentation in petechiae or purpura represents extravasation of blood into the skin. For this reason these lesions do not blanch on pressure. Purpura can be present with either a normal or decreased number of platelets. In infection, purpura is usually of the nonthrombocytopenic variety and is seen in many bacterial, viral, and rickettsial infections. The causes of nonthrombocytopenic purpura are not clearly understood, but suggested mechanisms include immune complex disease, actual infection of the vascular endothelium, and/or nonspecific capillary damage by the organism or its toxins. Infection may also be associated with thrombocytopenic purpura and may be either secondary to disseminated intravascular coagulation (DIC) or related to the direct effect of the microorganisms or its toxins on the circulating platelets.

Disseminated Intravascular Coagulation

DIC must be considered in any patient with fever and a decrease in platelets. It may occur in the early acute phase of any serious infection, especially with Gram-negative rod bacteremia or meningococcemia. DIC is characterized by intravascular consumption of platelets as well as other clotting factors. The consequences of this process are (a) a bleeding diathesis, (b) fibrinogen deposition in small vessels with resultant ischemic tissue damage, and (c) microangiopathic hemolytic anemia resulting from the damage to the red cell as it encounters the fibrin strands positioned across the lumina of small blood vessels.

The causes of DIC are diverse, but most cases are associated with severe infection (especially with endotoxemia), cancer, obstetrical problems, and the complications of surgery. A diagnosis of DIC is based on an evaluation of the peripheral smear, platelet count, bleeding time, prothrombin time, partial thromboplastin time, fibrinogen level, measurement of fibrin degradation products, and, if available, assay of clotting factors V and VIII.

The most effective therapy for DIC is successful management of the underlying predisposing illness. More controversial therapeutic modalities are sometimes employed, including the replacement of platelets or clotting factors and administration of anticoagulants such as heparin.

A related condition, purpura fulminans, is a similarly catastrophic disease, usually appearing in children in the convalescent phase of an infectious process.

Bacterial Endocarditis

Bacteremia and rickettsial infections account for the vast majority of treatable infections associated with petechiae. Among the bacteremic illnesses commonly associated with petechiae is bacterial endocarditis. This illness is often accompanied by small, red-brown, flat, and nonblanching lesions most frequently located on the extremities and mucous membranes, especially on the conjunctiva. The retina may demonstrate petechiae that are red with a white center (Roth spots). One must diligently search for petechiae all over the body, especially in the mouth, under the tongue, and on the tympanic membranes. Petechiae tend to appear in small crops and then fade in a few days, so that circling suspected lesions on the skin with a ballpoint pen and watching for their disappearance will help distinguish them from similar chronic spots on normal skin. The presence of petechiae in a febrile patient with known heart disease strongly suggests endocarditis. New or changing murmurs and the presence of heart failure, neurologic or renal dysfunction, or splenomegaly will add to the suspicion of endocarditis.

Meningococcemia

Bacteremias produced by neisseria organisms are also important causes of petechiae. Acute meningococcemia usually causes a rapidly progressing illness and must be recognized and treated immediately, for it can be fatal within hours. Fever and hypotension are dominant features of this disease, as are the skin manifestations. Typically, the early skin lesions are small, irregular, smudged, and raised, at times having a pustular center. The lesions are occasionally nodular and may be very tender. They occur on the extremities and trunk and may coalesce, forming large ecchymoses with areas of gangrene. However, this hemorrhagic rash is only one end of the spectrum; the early rash may be maculopapular and without a hemorrhagic component. Clinical evidence of meningitis may or may not be present in fulminant meningococcemia.

Frequently, kidney shaped Gram-negative diplococci are seen in smears of the skin lesions or of the buffy coat, especially within PMLs. When preparing a smear of petechiae, one should scrape the lesion with the dull end of a stylet and squeeze around it to produce exudation of clear serum. Using the sharp end of the stylet or a needle or scalpel blade may produce bleeding from the lesion, resulting in a slide of poor quality. A touch preparation of a drop of the serum is then made and Gram stained or stained with methylene blue if the Gram stain is nondiagnostic. Once a clinician strongly suspects meningococcemia, he must start treatment immediately. Meningococcemia is chronic in rare cases, with recurrent bouts of fever, polyarthritis, leukocytosis, and occasional skin lesions. This form of the disease is diagnosed by positive blood cultures.

Many patients with meningococcal infection present primarily with meningitis and not with fulminant meningococcemia. The finding of petechiae or other hemorrhagic lesions in a patient with fever, headaches, and stiff neck suggests meningococci as the etiology of the meningitis.

Gonococcemia

Disseminated gonococcal infection is a disease seen in sexually active individuals, especially females who are menstruating or pregnant. Fever and rash are common and are frequently associated with polyarthritis and tenosynovitis. The rash takes many forms, but usually begins as erythematous macules and papules and progresses to vesiculopustular lesions with a red base, which may at times become hemorrhagic. Smears of these lesions may reveal Gram-negative diplococci. The lesions are few in number and are much more common on the extremities than the trunk. They are frequently found on the extensor surfaces of the distal part of the extremities, especially near the joints. The skin lesions are often concentrated around the involved painful joints.

Other Bacteremias

Bacteremia caused by *P. aeruginosa* is seen especially in premature infants and patients who are debilitated, immunosuppressed, or suffering from extensive burns or leukemia. Pseudomonas bacteremia is almost never seen in normal individuals and is usually hospital-associated. Skin lesions are rare but, if present, may be helpful clues to the etiology. The lesions vary from painless maculopapular lesions on the trunk, resembling the rose spots of typhoid fever, to hemorrhagic papules or vesicles that may degenerate into painless necrotic ulcers ("ecthyma gangrenosum") and occur especially in the anogenital area or axillae. Subcutaneous nodules are also seen, rarely. Material aspirated from bullae and papules in pseudomonas septicemia demonstrates numerous organisms but few leukocytes. Biopsies show vasculitis with many organisms in the vessel walls. Cultures of these lesions and of the blood are usually positive. A rare acute enteric infection caused by pseudomonads, known as "Shanghai fever," may present with fever, diarrhea, headache, and rose spots.

Staphylococcemia and streptococcemia also may produce skin lesions. Staphylococcal bacteremia commonly results from infections of the skin or from indwelling IV catheters and may produce widespread metastatic pustules. At times petechial lesions are prominent. These metastatic skin lesions may occur with staphylococcal bacteremia whether or not endocarditis is present.

Streptococcal bacteremia is a problem in both the newborn and adult. In the latter, it usually originates from a cellulitis, a skin wound, or from a puerperal infection. The local site of entry of the streptococcus in a skin wound may be quite small and appear insignificant.

Many other bacterial species may cause bacteremia and petechiae. Less usual etiologies occur in patients predisposed by compromised immune status or by exposure to an environmental pathogen. Culture of blood and lesions is extremely important in such patients.

Rickettsial Infections

Rocky Mountain spotted fever (RMSF), or tick-borne typhus, characteristically produces a rash on the second to sixth day of illness. The rash begins as a fine eruption seen on the wrists, ankles, and forearms, and then extends to the palms and soles and may eventually involve the trunk and face. At first the rash is pink and maculopapular, fading on pressure. But after one to three days it can assume a deeper red color and become petechial. The mechanism for the petechiae in RMSF may involve leakage of blood through a damaged endothelium, as well as thrombocytopenia with or without DIC. Rarely, acral gangrene may supervene. The association of this rash with fever, extremely severe headache, and possible tick exposure warrants a presumptive diagnosis of RMSF, especially in the spring and summer in areas of the United States where the disease is endemic, e.g., the East coast, particularly the South Atlantic States.

It should be remembered that the early rash of RMSF may resemble rubeola. In the usual case of measles, however, the rash differs from RMSF by being more confluent and predominating on the face and trunk. The rash of rubella may also cause diagnostic confusion, but the rubella rash rarely becomes petechial, and the patient is infrequently as ill as a patient with RMSF. RMSF is sometimes confused with meningococcemia, but this latter disease is usually more fulminant, with the patient abruptly becoming ill and the rash appearing within hours of the onset of the illness. Also, the skin lesions of meningococcemia are frequently tender. Fortunately, treatment with chloramphenicol is satisfactory for both RMSF and meningococcemia, so when the differentiation cannot be made at the bedside, chloramphenicol is indicated and should be started immediately. In rare instances, viral infections, especially ECHO type 9, produce a petechial rash suggestive of meningococcemia or RMSF.

In the United States, Brill-Zinsser disease, or recrudescent louse-borne typhus, is seen occasionally among elderly patients from eastern Europe who had typhus many years before. In these patients the latent rickettsiae may become clinically evident once again, usually in a stressful situation such as during a postoperative period. The rash associated with this disease begins as a papular truncal eruption that spreads to the extremities and can become petechial.

Rat-Bite Fevers

Two other organisms that frequently produce skin lesions are the agents responsible for the rat-bite fevers. *Spirillum minus* infection starts with a maculopapular eruption on the abdomen, resembling the rose spots of typhoid. The bite site flares at the time that the symptomatic illness begins. The central rash may become petechial and spread to the extremities in an asymmetric manner, often including the palms and soles. The lesions are sparse but widespread. Joint involvement is occasionally present, and a relapsing course is frequent.

Streptobacillus moniliformis bacteremia may be secondary to either a rat bite or to ingestion of food contaminated by rodents. The illness produced is similar to *S. minus* infection, except that the incubation period is shorter in *S. moniliformis* infections (less than 10 days), and the rash, which is also maculopapular or petechial, is most extensive on the extremities, especially around the joints. The rash may become generalized. Joint involvement is quite common in this form of rat-bite fever. In the United States, laboratory workers represent a particularly high risk group.

MACULOPAPULAR RASHES

Rashes that are primarily maculopapular (macula = spot; papule = bump) with less likelihood of becoming petechial are seen in several important treatable infectious illnesses, including secondary syphilis, typhoid fever, mycoplasma, Lyme disease and several rickettsioses.

Secondary Syphilis

Secondary syphilis presents a characteristic syndrome of fever, generalized adenopathy, and a diffuse rash. This illness usually becomes clinically overt between two weeks to six months following the primary chancre. The rash, which in moist areas is teeming with spirochetes, may take any form except vesicular. Usually it is macular, papular or maculopapular. White patients tend to have maculopapular lesions, while nonwhites more often demonstrate papules, frequently with annular or circinate patterns. The rash is nearly always generalized, usually including the palms and soles. The rash is neither painful nor pruritic. Mucous patches or condylomata lata when seen are highly characteristic of this infection.

Rickettsial Diseases

Rickettsial disease frequently begins with a macular rash. As described above, RMSF may cause a faint pink macular rash suggestive of measles that may or may not progress to petechiae. Murine typhus, transmitted by the rat flea, is seen mainly in the southern half of the United States and is a milder illness than RMSF, with moderate headache, chills, and fever. Rash is present in only one-half the cases and appears on about the fifth day of illness. It begins in the axillae and inner surface of the arms, but then may quickly become more generalized. It is most dramatic on the trunk, being less prominent on the face, extremities, palms, and soles. The rash is macular or maculopapular and only very rarely petechial. These clinical features help distinguish this rash from that seen in RMSF. Ehrlichiosis is a tick-borne infection that resembles RMSF, with fever, headache and myalgias. Most patients with ehrlichiosis have no rash, but when a rash appears it may include palms and soles and occasionally produce a generalized erythema. *R. conorii* (tick typhus), seen in travelers returning from Africa or the Mediterranean basin, also is a rickettsial infection resembling RMSF. The rash is maculopapular but may be petechial or vesicular and include trunk, extremities and face. Classic epidemic typhus caused by *R. prowazekii*, is being seen rarely in the USA from a reservoir in flying squirrels. The rash of typhus progresses from the trunk to the extremities and tends to spare the face, palms and soles. It may be petechial in severe infection. The relapse of typhus, Brill-Zinsser disease, is mentioned above. It is a milder, though similar, illness, and may produce macules or petechiae.

Typhoid Fever

Typhoid fever has protean presentations, including fever, prostration, leukopenia, abdominal pain, splenomegaly, constipation, and at times, relative bradycardia. A most helpful clinical clue when present is the detection of rose spots. These spots are slightly raised pink papules that blanch on pressure. They develop in crops of 10 to 20 lesions and are found on the upper abdomen, lower chest, and midback. Smears, cultures, and biopsies of these lesions may reveal the organisms. Usually, rose spots make their appearance during the second week of illness, when the abdominal pain begins. Then, over the next two to three weeks, other new crops emerge. Although rose spots are seen very rarely in enteric fever due to other salmonella species, when present, they may be more extensive and involve the face and limbs as well as the trunk.

Psittacosis

Horder's spots, which resemble the rose spots of typhoid fever, may be seen in patients with psittacosis. These patients usually have myalgias and severe headache and frequently demonstrate pneumonia and splenomegaly. Epidemiologic history is crucial because the disease is usually acquired from birds, especially turkeys, parrots, and parakeets. Infection may be transmitted either by sick birds or birds that are convalescent carriers.

Mycoplasma

Mycoplasma infection usually produces atypical pneumonia in a child or young adult. Headaches, nonproductive cough and myalgias are common. Rash frequently accompanies the infection and may be of many varieties, including maculopapular. A clue to mycoplasmal infection is the long incubation period, usually two to three weeks, between exposure to a contact and the onset of illness.

Lyme Disease

Lyme disease begins as erythema chronicum migrans two to three weeks after the tick bite. Systemic signs are common (fever, malaise, headaches) and the skin lesions are multiple in 10 to 15 percent of patients. Although the classic ECM is an expanding erythematous round area with central clearing, secondary lesions are smaller and lack an indurated center. If untreated, ECM will clear, but patients are at risk for later development of cardiac, neurologic and rheumatologic sequelae.

VESICULAR/BULLOUS OR PUSTULAR RASH

A vesicular or pustular rash may occur in an acutely ill patient. Staphylococcemia and gonococcemia, already discussed, are important causes of this syndrome, as they may cause widespread metastatic skin infection. Another treatable disease causing a vesicular eruption is rickettsialpox. After being bitten by a mite, the patient develops a painless pustular lesion at the bite site. This lesion then forms a black eschar. The patient feels well at this stage of the illness, but then develops fever and generalized constitutional signs. During this latter phase of the disease, a generalized maculopapular rash appears, with each papule becoming capped by a firm vesicle. These lesions differ from those of varicella, which are completely transformed into vesicles and not merely capped by them. *R. conorii*, described above, may produce a pustular eruption also.

Disseminated *Herpes simplex* infection also presents as a generalized vesicular rash. It occurs only rarely in normal adults, being seen primarily in newborns and in patients with altered host defenses. Varicella causes a characteristic rash with vesicles on an erythematous base occurring at all stages of development (new, maturing and crusting). The lesions are concentrated on the trunk and involve the scalp and axillae and the skin behind the ears. Adults are at risk for pneumonia when they develop varicella. Herpes zoster infection may, in patients with poor host defenses, become generalized rather than remaining localized to a specific dermatome. Zoster immune globulin may be given prophylactically if exposure to *Varicella-zoster* virus has occurred less than 48 hours before. *Vibrio vulnificus* bacteremia is acquired by ingestion of undercooked seafood and is a risk for patients with underlying liver or renal disease or diabetes. Skin lesions are common and frequently develop into hemorrhagic bullae.

Diffuse Erythemas

Diffuse erythematous eruptions may be caused by a variety of infections. Group A streptococci can cause scarlet fever, a syndrome of pharyngitis and diffuse erythema with varying degrees of organ dysfunction. The erythema is finely punctate and blanching, but may become petechial in skin folds in the axillary and antecubital areas (Pastia's lines). Concentration in the upper trunk, circumoral pallor, and swollen red papillae on the tongue ("strawberry tongue") are characteristics of the scarlet fever exanthem. An associated enanthem of the soft and hard palate is generally demonstrable. Elevation at the site of hair follicles produces a "sandpaper" sensation on palpation, a helpful finding in dark-skinned patients. Desquamation, especially of hands and feet and groin, is commonly seen in convalescence.

Group A streptococci also cause a toxic-shock-like illness, with hypotension and multi-organ failure. Usually, localized soft tissue infection is evident, characterized by localized pain, swelling and erythema; this focal infection frequently represents myositis or faciitis and requires urgent debridement. Less commonly, generalized erythema is the predominant manifestation. Streptococcal pyrogenic exotoxins A, B, and C are the cause of this syndrome and of scarlet fever.

Staphylococcus aureus is the cause of classic toxic shock syndrome, manifested by fever, hypotension and multiple organ dysfunction. The staphylococci may be causing clinically-evident infection or simply colonizing. The cause of the syndrome is one of a variety of toxins (TSST-1, enterotoxin B or C). A related staphylococcal syndrome is staph scalded skin syndrome (SSSS), a painful erythroderma caused by epidermolysins A and B. Superficial

TABLE 6.2. CELLULITIS—ETIOLOGY

Most patients:	Strep, Staph
Additional Considerations:	Diabetes—Gram ⊖ bacilli Compromised host—fungi Human bite—Eikinella Dog/cat bite—Pasturella multocida Tick bite—Lyme disease Fresh water—aeromonas Salt water—vibrio Fish, animal products—erysipelothrix Animals—campylobacter

TABLE 6.3. ULCERATING LESIONS—DIAGNOSIS

	Stain	Culture	Serologic Test
Amebiasis	x		
Anthrax	x	x	
Blastomycosis	x	x	
Diphtheria	x	x	
Ecthyma (staphylococcal, streptococcal)	x	x	
Herpes simplex	x	x	
Leishmaniasis	x		
Melioidosis		x	
M. hemophilum		x	
M. marinum		x	
M. ulcerans		x	
Nocardiosis	x	x	
Sporotrichosis	x	x	
Schistosoma cutis	x		
Syphilis	x		x
Tuberculosis		x	
Tularemia		x	x

sloughing of the skin may occur (Nicolsky's sign) due to involvement of the granular layer of the epidermis. This syndrome occurs in children; a similar entity, toxic epidermal necrolysis (TEN) occurs in adults, affects the dermal-epidermal junction, and usually results from a drug reaction.

Kawasaki disease, or mucocutaneous lymph node syndrome, occurs in children under the age of five. It resembles scarlet fever, but streptococcal infection is not present, and antibiotics have no effect. Coronary arteritis occurs and is responsible for the occasional fatality seen.

Ehrlichiosis is a rickettsial infection that usually resembles mild RMSF, but may be associated with fever, multi-organ involvement, hypotension and erythema, i.e., a toxic-shock-like syndrome. *S. viridans* bacteremia has been associated with chemotherapy-induced damage to oral and gastrointestinal mucosa and may produce generalized erythema. Finally, *Arcanobacterium (Corynebacterium) hemolyticum* is a cause of pharyngitis in teenagers and young adults that may be complicated by a diffuse erythematous eruption.

URTICARIAL RASH

Most infectious causes of urticarial eruptions are not specifically treatable (Table 6.1), but two important exceptions are mycoplasmal infection and Lyme disease, both described above.

As noted previously, this chapter covers generalized eruptions, or rashes. However, localized infectious skin lesions are important and closely related entities, and are presented in tabular form as "Cellulitis" (Table 6.2) and "Ulcerating Lesions" (Table 6.3).

Drug Reactions

It is important to remember that drug reactions can mimic all of the rashes discussed above. The occurrence of a rash in a febrile patient receiving antibiotic therapy may be confusing, since the rash could be either drug-induced or part of the illness for which the drug is being given. Rickettsial infections may be particularly troublesome in this regard, because the rash may appear after several days of treatment with antibiotics and thereby lead the clinician to misinterpret the rash as a drug reaction, rather than as support for the diagnosis of rickettsial disease. In patients with infectious mononucleosi, a maculopapular eruption occurs almost universally if ampicillin is given. This rash represents an interaction between drug and disease process and is not thought to be allergic in nature; the pathogenesis remains unexplained, however.

Allergic reactions and other noninfectious causes of rash are listed in Table 6.4.

TABLE 6.4. NONINFECTIOUS CAUSES OF RASH

Petechial/Purpura/ Purpuric Vesicles	Maculopapular	Vesicle/ Bullae/ Pustules	Urticarial Eruption	Erythema
Allergy	Allergy	Allergy	Allergy	Allergy
Hypercoagulatable states	Erythema multiforme	Plant dermatitis	Vasculitis	Vasodilation
Low platelets of any cause	Erythema marginatum	Pemphigus	Malignancy	Eczema
Scurvy		Porphyria cutanea tarda	Idiopathic	Psoriasis
Henoch-Schonlein purpura	Systemic lupus erythematosis			Lymphoma
Palpable purpura	Dermatomyositis	Erythema multiforme bullosum		Pityriosis rubra
(Hypersensitivity vasculitis)	Serum sickness			Sezary's syndrome
Acute rheumatic fever				
Hyperglobulinemia				
Amyloidosis				
Systemic lupus erythematosis				

DIFFERENTIAL DIAGNOSIS OF INFECTIOUS DISEASES

TABLE 6.5. DIAGNOSTIC CHART: RASH—SELECTED ETIOLOGIES

Disease	Epidemiology/Pathogenesis	Clinical Signs
A. Bacteremia		
1. Bacterial endocarditis	Acute: Patient may not have history of significant valvular heart disease. Frequently associated with bacteremia with *S. aureus,* but at times with enterococci or with Gram-negative rods. Drug addicts are at high risk. Lesions are usually tricuspid, but left-sided involvement is common. Subacute: Patients with rheumatic, arteriosclerotic or congenital heart disease, often after bacteremia with organisms of low virulence. Prosthetic: Patients with prosthetic heart valves are also at very high risk, both at time of surgery and with bacteremia after surgery.	Fever, anemia, splenomegaly, new or changing murmur, Roth spots, splinters, hemorrhages, petechiae, and Osler's nodes. Deterioration in cardiac, CNS, or renal status. Changes may be very subtle.
2. Meningococcemia	Organisms harbored subclinically in nasopharynx, illness at times preceded by pharyngitis.	Fever, prostration, hypotension; meningismus may be present. Patient severely ill.

Rash	Diagnosis	Initial Treatment (Alternate Rx is in Parentheses)
Small petechial lesions on the skin and mucous membranes should be searched for carefully.	Blood cultures are positive in 85% if 5 separate specimens are drawn; more than 5 have small additional yield. Positive rheumatoid factor in 50% of patients who have had disease longer than 6 weeks. Low serum complement if nephritis present. Most common lab abnormality is elevated ESR. If blood cultures are negative; perform fungal and Q fever serologies; inoculate small amounts of blood to dilute serum antibody, do buffy coat smear, stain ear lobe histocytes, culture for cell-wall deficient organisms, and discuss with the microbiologist any additional media or cultural techniques that could be attempted. If embolectomy performed, stain and culture material obtained for bacteria and fungi.	Depends on specific organisms isolated. If therapy begun before specific organism has been isolated, use the following combination of antibiotics: *Acute:* Nafcillin or vancomycin + gentamicin. *Subacute:* ampicillin + gentamicin (vancomycin and gentamicin). *Prosthetic value:* Vancomycin and gentamicin ± Rifampin.
Petechiae that are irregular, raised, and frequently tender on the trunk and extremities. May become ecchymotic. Neck and face usually spared. Rash may progress in minutes or hours.	Gram stain of buffy coat. Smear and culture of petechiae. Blood cultures. CSF smear and culture. Studies for DIC indicated.	Penicillin G (third-generation cephalosporin).

(continued)

TABLE 6.5. (continued) **DIAGNOSTIC CHART: RASH—SELECTED ETIOLOGIES**

Disease	Epidemiology/Pathogenesis	Clinical Signs
3. Gonococcemia	Epidemiology similar to that of localized gonococcal infections, i.e., venereal spread. Frequently the source of the bacteremia is asymptomatic.	Seen especially in sexually active females menstruating or at term; see fever, polyarthritis, and tenosynovitis, which after several days may localize in one or two joints. Patients usually only moderately ill.
4. Pseudomonas septicemia	Patients receiving antibiotics, premature infants, the debilitated and immunosuppressed, burn patients, leukemia patients in relapse. Pseudomonas colonizes patients from moist environment such as nebulizers.	Fever, prostration, hypotension in the appropriate host. Usually occurs in hospitalized patients.
5. Staphylococcal bacteremia	Associated with catheters, skin lesions, parenteral drug abuse, wound infection.	Fever, prostration, severe myalgia. Endocarditis occurs frequently with sustained staphylococcal bacteremia. Multiple sites of metastatic infection may be present such as multiple pulmonary and/or brain abscesses.
6. Streptococcal bacteremia	Seen in newborns or in adults with cellulitis, other skin infections, or puerperal sepsis.	Fever, prostration.

Rash	Diagnosis	Initial Treatment (Alternate Rx is in Parentheses)
A few scattered erythematous macules, papules, and petechiae, which may progress to vesicopustules and finally hemorrhagic lesions. More on extremities than trunk, frequently around inflamed joints.	Blood cultures. Smear and culture of joint fluid, skin lesions, urethra. Culture cervix, rectum, and pharynx.	Third-generation cephalosporin.
Lesions infrequently seen, but helpful when present. Vary from painless maculopapules to hemorrhagic vesicles, which may progress to necrotic ulcers in axilla or anogenital area.	Blood cultures. Smear and culture of materials aspirated from bullae and papules or from skin biopsy. Green fluorescence of urine, from verdoglobinuria, is helpful in diagnosis of severe pseudomonas infection in burn patients.	Tobramycin, amikacin, or gentamicin in combination with ticarcillin or piperacillin.
Disseminated pustular rash, at times petechial.	Blood cultures. Buffy coat smear. Smear and culture of skin lesions. Teichoic acid antibodies may be present.	Vancomycin.
Petechial.	Blood cultures. Buffy coat smear. Smear and culture lesions.	Penicillin G (cefazolin).

(continued)

TABLE 6.5. (continued) DIAGNOSTIC CHART: RASH—SELECTED ETIOLOGIES

Disease	Epidemiology/Pathogenesis	Clinical Signs
B. Rocky Mountain spotted fever	Most common in Southeast U.S., but seen in most regions. The rickettsia are spread by tick bite. Usually seen in warmer months of the year.	Fever, and severe headache, followed by rash 2–6 days later.
C. Rat-bite fever (*S. minus*)	Rat bite.	Fever, polyarthritis. Bite site flares when acute illness begins.
D. Rat-bite fever (*S. moniliformis*)	Rat bite or infected food.	Fever, polyarthritis. No flare at bite site when illness begins. In fact, bite site may not be obvious.
E. Rickettsialpox	Spread by bite of mite.	Bite develops into eschar; then patient develops fever and rash. Patients usually not extremely sick.
F. Secondary syphilis	Sexually transmitted. Onset generally 2 weeks to 6 months after primary.	Fever; generalized, nontender lymphadenopathy.

Rash	Diagnosis	Initial Treatment (Alternate Rx is in Parentheses)
Early rash is pink, macular, and blanches, resembling measles or drug eruption; it later becomes petechial. Wrists and ankles are first involved, followed by palms and soles; rash may finally progress centripetally to trunk and face.	Serology helpful, but treatment should be begun on basis of history and physical exam. Thrombocytopenia common. DIC may be seen. Organisms may be seen in biopsy of petechiae by trained observer and can be readily seen with immunofluorescent staining.	Doxycycline (chloramphenicol).
Maculopapular rash on abdomen progressing to extremities and becoming petechial; may involve palms and soles.	Inoculate blood or wound aspirate into mice or guinea pigs. Dark field of bite, rash, or node aspirate. False-positive VDRL.	Penicillin G (doxycycline).
Maculopapular or petechial; most extensive on extremities, especially around joints; may become generalized.	Culture blood, wound, joint. Serology helpful.	Penicillin G (doxycycline).
Generalized, maculopapular; then each papule becomes topped by a vesicle.	Serology helpful.	Tetracycline (chloramphenicol).
Maculopapular (especially in white patients), papular (especially in non-white patients), or pustular. Usually, rash is generalized and includes palms and soles, but may occasionally be confined to face or to palms and soles. Rash is not pruritic or painful.	Dark-field of moist areas of rash; VDRL and FTA-ABS nearly always positive in secondary syphilis.	Penicillin (doxycycline).

(continued)

TABLE 6.5. (continued) DIAGNOSTIC CHART: RASH—SELECTED ETIOLOGIES

Disease	Epidemiology/Pathogenesis	Clinical Signs
G. Murine typhus	Transmitted by the rat flea. Seen occasionally in the southern U.S.	Headache, chills, fever.
H. Typhoid fever	In the U.S. the source of contamination is usually the stool of elderly chronic carriers. The organism can be spread by contaminated food, water; flies can be vectors from feces or food.	Headaches, fever, cramps, constipation, cough, epistaxis, leukopenia, splenomegaly, and bradycardia. Diarrhea may be present at times rather than constipation. Pulse-temperature dissociation sometimes a helpful clue.
DIC	Any severe infection, but most frequently due to Gram-negative rod bacteremia and meningococcemia. Pneumococcal bacteremia may be complicated by DIC, especially in patients with absent or poorly functioning spleen.	May have widespread bleeding tendencies.
R. Conorii	Seen in Africa and Mediterranean basin.	Fever, headache, myalgias.
Mycoplasma	Respiratory pathogen, long incubation period (weeks).	Fever, headache, non-productive cough; other organ systems frequently involved.

Rash	Diagnosis	Initial Treatment (Alternate Rx is in Parentheses)
Rash is maculopapular. It begins in axillae and inner surface of arms, quickly becomes generalized, most intense on trunk, limited on face, extremities, palms, and soles. Rash is not always present or obvious in this illness.	Serology helpful but treatment should be initiated on basis of strong clinical suspicion.	Doxycycline (chloramphenicol).
Rose spots are seen in only 10% of patients, but are helpful when present; slightly raised pink papules, which blanch on pressure. They blossom in crops of 10–20 lesions and are found on the trunk, anteriorly and posteriorly.	Culture blood, urine, and stool. Mononuclear cells in stool smear if diarrhea present. Smear and culture rose spots. Bone marrow culture at times very helpful. Serology helpful.	Depending on sensitivities, may use ciprofloxacin, TMP-SMX, or ceftriaxone. Some still prefer chloramphenicol.
Petechiae, ecchymoses.	Decreased platelets. Schistocytes present. Decrease in fibrinogen, factors V and VIII. Increased fibrin split products. Falling ESR. Prolonged PT, PTT, and bleeding and clotting time.	Treat underlying disease. (Heparin has not been shown to be very effective in this setting but is sometimes used).
Usually maculo-papular, but may be petechial and rarely vesiculo-pustular.	Specific stain of skin biopsy; serology.	Doxycycline.
Maculopapular most common but also see other forms, including urticarial.	Serology.	Doxycycline or erythromycin.

(continued)

TABLE 6.5. (continued) DIAGNOSTIC CHART: RASH—SELECTED ETIOLOGIES

Disease	Epidemiology/Pathogenesis	Clinical Signs
Lyme disease	Transmitted by bite of ixodes tick. Rash result of skin infection with borrelia.	Erythema chronicum migrans, often associated with fever, headache, "flu-like illness."
Varicella	Respiratory route, may contact from pt. with zoster, if susceptible.	Fever, malaise, thrombocytopenia and pneumonia in adult.
Kawasaki Disease	Children <5.	Coronary arteritis, fever, cervical adenopathy, skin and mucous membrane involvement.
S. viridans bacteremia	Chemotherapy–induced damage to oral & GI mucosa.	Hypotension on multi-organ involvement.
C. hemolyticum	Teenagers and young adults.	Sore throat.
Ehrlichiosis	Tick bite. ?Dog contact.	Fever, headache, myalgias; most patients have no rash.
Staphylococcus aureus	SSSS-infection by strain producing epidermolysin.	No significant toxicity.
	TSS-colonization or infection by strain producing TSST-1, enterotoxins B or C.	Fever, ↓ BP, multi-organ failure.

Rash	Diagnosis	Initial Treatment (Alternate Rx is in Parentheses)
Classically a single expanding red spot with clearing center. But may be multiple, and center may not clear or may become vesicular or necrotic.	Clinical suspicion, serology.	Doxycycline.
Vesicles on red base. Centripetal concentrations, lesions of all ages in same site. Scalp and axilla and skin behind ears.	Clinical, Tzanck prep, biopsy.	Acyclovir.
Erythema, swelling of hands & feet, conjunctival suffusion, mucous membrane involvement.	Clinical, exclusion of other etiologies, e.g., strep.	IV gamma-globulin, ASA.
Diffuse erythema.	Culture.	Penicillin.
Diffuse erythema.	Culture.	Erythromycin.
Usually maculo-papular, but petechiae or diffuse erythema may be seen.	Serology. Leukocyte inclusions. PCR.	Doxycycline.
Painful erythoderma. Nicolsky's sign.	Clinical, culture.	Nafcillin.
Diffuse erythema, mucous membranes involved. Late desquamation.	Clinical, culture.	Nafcillin.

(continued)

TABLE 6.5. (continued) DIAGNOSTIC CHART: RASH—SELECTED ETIOLOGIES

Disease	Epidemiology/Pathogenesis	Clinical Signs
Streptococcus pyogenes	Scarlet fever: SPE A, B, C.	Pharyngitis.
	TSS: SPE A, B, C. May follow minor trauma.	Localized soft tissue infection with ↓ BP, multi-organ failure.
Vibrio vulnificus	Ingestion of undercooked seafood. A risk in patients with diabetes, liver, or renal dysfunction. Also may cause wound infection by direct contamination by seawater.	Septicemia, minimal G-I symptoms, wound infection, extremely painful.

Rash	Diagnosis	Initial Treatment (Alternate Rx is in Parentheses)
Scarlet fever-generalized punctute erythema, bleeding into skin lines; circumoral pallor.	Clinical, culture.	Penicillin.
Usually localized erythema & edema, but erythema may be generalized.	Clinical, culture, CT scan.	Debridement. Penicillin; some would add clindamycin.
Cellulitis, hemorrhagic bullae, lymphangitis.	Clinical, culture.	Debridement, doxycycline plus aminoglycoside.

7

MONOARTHRITIS

Most organisms that cause monoarthritis can also produce polyarthritis. However, there are a few infectious processes that typically involve only one joint (Table 7.1).

BACTERIAL ETIOLOGY

By far the most common etiology of an infectious monoarthritis is bacterial. The bacteria may invade the joint from the bloodstream, by direct extension from an adjacent infection in bone or soft tissues, or from iatrogenic introduction by a contaminated needle. The clinical presentation is characterized by fever, leukocytosis, and an extremely painful joint. Frequently the affected joint is swollen and tender, and the overlying skin is erythematous.

Children have a particularly high incidence of septic arthritis. In this younger age group, the most frequent organism found is *S. aureus*, followed by beta-hemolytic streptococci, pneumococci, *H. influenzae*, and Gram-negative rods. *H. influenzae* is a particularly important cause from six months to two years of age.

Gonococci are the organisms most frequently associated with monoarthritis in adults, followed by staphylococci, pneumococci,

TABLE 7.1. MONOARTHRITIS

A. Bacterial[a]
  1. Adults
     a. Gonococcus
     b. Staphylococcus
     c. Pneumococcus
     d. Streptococcus
     e. Others
  2. Children
     a. Staphylococcus
     b. Streptococcus
     c. Pneumococcus
     d. H. influenza
     e. Gram-negative rods
     f. Others

B. Tuberculosis

C. Fungal
  1. *B. dermatitidis*
  2. *C. immitis*
  3. Others

D. Rare etiologies (usually polyarticular and discussed in chapter 8): Lyme disease, syphilis, HIV, hepatitis B and other viruses.

[a] Most common cause.

and streptococci. Gonococcal monoarthritis is seen primarily in young, sexually active patients, especially women, and frequently follows a bout of polyarthritis before the localization in one or two joints. Tenosynovitis may accompany the joint inflammation, as may skin lesions that include macules, petechiae, and vesiculopustules. These findings are very characteristic of gonococcal infection.

When Gram-positive cocci are the cause of monoarthritis, the underlying source of the dissemination is sometimes evident. For example, when arthritis develops in a patient with pneumococcal pneumonia, it is most likely secondary to pneumococcal bacteremia, whereas a septic joint in a patient with a staphylococcal skin abscess suggests a staphylococcal etiology for the arthritis.

Gram-negative rods and Candida are additional causes of septic monoarthritis in immunocompromised patients and IV drug abusers. In the latter group of patients, unusual sites of involvement are common and include the vertebral, sternoclavicular, and costochondral joints.

Since there are few features that distinguish one cause of bacterial joint infection from another, Gram stain and culture of joint fluid are essential for etiologic diagnosis. Blood cultures are positive in up to 25 percent of cases, and at times the blood is the only site from which the organism can be recovered. In more severe disseminated infections, multiple joints may become involved, and the frequency of positive blood cultures is greater.

The x-ray findings in septic arthritis are usually normal; abnormalities are seen only several weeks after infection has occurred. Thus in acute infections, except for nonspecific soft tissue swelling, x-rays are less likely to be as helpful as in chronic infections such as tuberculosis or fungal disease.

TUBERCULOUS ARTHRITIS

Arthritis caused by *M. tuberculosis* is usually secondary to tuberculous osteomyelitis, but it can be primary. It is characterized by the insidious onset of joint pain and swelling. Usually a single weight-bearing joint is affected, frequently following trauma to the joint. The usual age of onset is during the first three decades of life, and constitutional symptoms may be minimal to absent. The most common site of involvement is the spine. Narrowing of the intervertebral space is seen on x-ray, with destruction of adjacent vertebral bodies resulting in the spine settling forward and a characteristic deformity (the "gibbus"). An abscess may then form in the muscles around the spine, e.g., the psoas muscle.

The presence of pulmonary and other extrapulmonary tuberculosis is not always apparent. However, if the PPD is negative and the patient is not anergic, tuberculosis is unlikely. The diagnosis of tuberculous arthritis is established by finding the organism on smear or culture of joint fluid, synovial biopsy, or contiguous bone (if osteomyelitis is present). The presence of caseating granulomas without demonstration of the organism is characteristic of tuberculosis. It is also noteworthy that atypical mycobacteria are recognized as rare causes of arthritis.

LESS COMMON ETIOLOGIES

Fungi, too, may cause an infectious monoarthritis. *Blastomyces dermatitidis* may cause a monoarthritis by invading the joint from a neighboring osteomyelitic focus. Other fungi, such as *Coccidioides immitis*, may also cause a septic monoarthritis, but are more likely to involve multiple joints.

Most other organisms can cause septic monoarthritis, although the organisms mentioned above account for the vast majority of infections of a single joint. Some infections cause monoarthritis on occasion, but are more likely to produce inflammation in multiple joints and are therefore discussed in the next chapter (polyarthritis). These include Lyme disease, syphilis, and viral infection such as hepatitis B and HIV infection.

An important entity to remember is the superimposition of a septic process on joints that are already damaged by noninfectious diseases. Any damaged joint is more susceptible to infection. Furthermore, patients with underlying joint disease may have an infected joint during a flare-up of their chronic disease, and the signs and symptoms of pyogenic infection may be misinterpreted. For example, rheumatoid disease is the underlying arthritis most commonly complicated by pyogenic joint infection. Clues to the presence of infection in one of the many joints involved by the rheumatoid process include disproportionate inflammation of a single joint and failure of the infected joint or joints to respond to therapy directed at the rheumatoid arthritis. A Gram stain and culture of the aspirated joint fluid is imperative, since the cell counts and glucose level in the joint fluid of patients with rheumatoid arthritis may closely resemble the findings in septic arthritis.

Gout is another form of arthritis that may simulate infectious arthritis or predispose to a septic joint. If there is any doubt concerning the diagnosis or if therapy for gout is ineffective, appropriate joint fluid studies, including Gram stain and culture, are indicated in addition to a search for urate crystals. In addition to gout, other diseases that cause monoarthritis may resemble infection or be complicated by infection; these are presented in Table 7.2.

TABLE 7.2. NONINFECTIOUS MONOARTHRITIS

A. Gout, pseudogout

B. Rheumatoid arthritis (especially juvenile rheumatoid arthritis)

C. Trauma

D. Tumors

E. Hemarthrosis

F. Osteochondritis

G. Palindromic rheumatism

H. Pigmented villonodular synovitis

TABLE 7.3. DIAGNOSTIC CHART: INFECTIOUS MONOARTHRITIS—SELECTED ETIOLOGIES

Disease	Joint Fluid[a]	Diagnosis	Initial Treatment
A. Infectious			
1. Bacterial arthritis	Group III.	Gram stain and culture of joint fluid; blood culture. If gonococcal etiology is suspected, obtain additional cultures from rectum, throat, and cervix, and Gram stain and culture urethra and skin lesions. In addicts and immunocompromised patients, beware of Gram-negative rods and fungal infection as well as staphylococcal infection.	Before culture report is available, treatment depends on Gram-stain result. If Gram stain shows no organism, the therapy is selected on basis of patient's age, underlying disease, and evidence of other sites of infection (see text).
2. Tuberculous	Group II or III.	AFB stain and culture of synovial biopsy (best) or synovial fluid; PPD; pulmonary TB present in approximately ½ of cases.	Isoniazid, pyrazinamide, ethambutol, and rifampin.
3. Fungal arthritis (limited data available)	Group I or II. May be bloody.	Fungal culture and stains of joint fluid and of synovial biopsy; serologic tests helpful. Frequently other organ systems are involved.	Amphotericin B.
B. Noninfectious			
1. Gout	Group II. Urate crystals present, demonstrating negative birefringence.	Characteristic crystals in joint fluid; fever and leukocytosis may be present. Other evidence of gout; chronic joint disease, tophi, etc. Response to colchicine is characteristic. X-ray findings may be suggestive.	Colchicine; anti-inflammatory therapy.

(continued)

TABLE 7.3. *(continued)* **DIAGNOSTIC CHART: INFECTIOUS MONOARTHRITIS—SELECTED ETIOLOGIES**

Disease	Joint Fluid[a]	Diagnosis	Initial Treatment
2. Pseudogout	Group II. Rarely count reaches 100,000–200,000; calcium pyrophosphate crystals in joint fluid, demonstrating positive birefringence.	Characteristic crystals in joint fluid; fever and leukocytosis may be present. Chondrocalcinosis on x-ray of involved joints.	Anti-inflammatory therapy.
3. Rheumatoid arthritis	Group II. Glucose may be decreased. Complement may be decreased.	Rheumatoid factor in serum in 80% of patients. Antinuclear antibody. Cholesterol crystals in joint fluid. Joint x-rays may show characteristic changes. Beware of bacterial suprainfections.	Anti-inflammatory therapy.
4. Trauma	Group I. May have moderate number of RBCs.	History; other signs of trauma.	Symptomatic therapy.
5. Osteoarthritis	Group I.	Age of patient; absence of systemic symptomatology, characteristic x-ray changes.	Symptomatic therapy.

[a] Joint Fluid Types

	WNL	Noninflammatory Group I	Inflammatory Group II	Purulent Group III
WBC/mm^3	<50	<3000	3000–50,000	50,000–300,000
% PMN	<25	<25	>70	>90
Volume (ml)	<4	>4	>4	>4
Color	Clear/yellow	Yellow	Yellow-white	White
Clarity	Transparent	Transparent	Transparent-opaque	Opaque
Viscosity	Good	Fair	Poor	Very poor
Glucose	= serum	= serum	= serum	<50% of serum glucose

Adapted from McCarty, Lea & Febiger, ed #12 p. 65

8

POLYARTHRITIS

Many important infectious diseases include polyarthritis among their cardinal manifestations. Arthralgias are so common and ill-defined as to be nonspecific. Therefore, in the following discussion, only those infectious diseases associated with polyarthritis, i.e., objectively inflamed joints, will be considered. For purposes of differential diagnosis, a few of the most common noninfectious causes of polyarthritis are included in this discussion.

Many of the processes that usually cause a polyarthritis sometimes present as a monoarthritis. For this reason, the chapters discussing polyarthritis and monoarthritis should be reviewed together in the workup of a patient with arthritis suspected to be infectious in etiology.

The most common infectious causes of polyarthritis are bacterial (any bacteremia, particularly gonococcemia, or bacterial endocarditis), and viral, especially rubella, mumps, and the hepatitis syndrome (Table 8.1).

Gonococcal Arthritis

The gonococcus is the most frequent infectious cause of both polyarthritis and monoarthritis in the adult. Gonococcal arthritis is

TABLE 8.1. POLYARTHRITIS

Common Etiologies	Rare Etiologies
Bacterial infections	
Gonococcemia[a]	Typhoid fever
Subacute bacterial endocarditis[a]	Brucellosis
Meningococcemia	Cat scratch disease
S. moniliformis	
Most other bacteremias	
Viral infections	
Hepatitis prodrome[a]	EBV infection
Rubella[a]	Influenza
Mumps	Arbovirus
Parvovirus B19	Hepatitis A
HIV	
Spirochetal infections	
Secondary syphilis	
S. minus (rat-bite fever)	
Lyme disease	
Fungal infections	
Coccidioidomycosis	
Chlamydial infections	
Lymphogranuloma venereum	
Miscellaneous	
Reiter's Disease	M. pneumoniae infections
Whipple's Disease	Filariasis
"Reactive" arthritis	
Rheumatic Fever	

[a] Most common causes.

an important infectious cause of polyarthritis, especially in the young, sexually active female. Dissemination of the gonococcus from the genital source frequently occurs during menstruation or pregnancy. Clinical evidence of localized gonococcal infection may or may not be present, since cervical infections in the female are usually asymptomatic. However, a careful search for localized gonococcal infection in the cervix, urethra, rectum, or pharynx should always be made. A variety of skin lesions occur, especially on the extensor surface of the extremity around inflamed joints. The most common skin manifestations are vesiculopustular lesions which may show typical intracellular Gram-negative diplococci when appropriately smeared. Cultures from these skin lesions are usually negative. A very useful clinical clue in this form of arthritis is the finding of tenosynovitis, as well as inflammation of the joint itself. Often an acute polyarthritis with positive blood cultures is followed in several days by a monoarthritis with negative blood cultures and positive joint fluid cultures.

Meningococcemia

As with gonococcemia, acute meningococcemia may produce a polyarthritis. In addition, the rare chronic form of meningococcemia may mimic gonococcemia with its periodic bouts of fever, petechiae, and ecchymoses. Resolution without therapy may occur, but the disease should be treated with appropriate antibiotics, since a more fulminant form of meningococcemia may occur at any time. Also, meningococcal meningitis is occasionally complicated by a sterile large joint polyarthritis long after therapy is begun.

Reiter's Syndrome

Another disease that may be of infectious etiology and may closely resemble gonococcal arthritis is Reiter's syndrome. This entity consists of the triad of conjunctivitis, urethritis, and arthritis, often occurring after sexual exposure or a bout of diarrhea. Commonly, only one or two of these findings are present. Unlike gonococcal arthritis, Reiter's syndrome is seen almost exclusively in males. Furthermore, the classical rash of Reiter's syndrome, keratoderma blennorrhagica, though not pathognomonic, is very distinctive, consisting of violaceous papules appearing on the palms and soles and associated with hyperkeratosis. Aortic insufficiency may rarely complicate Reiter's syndrome and may cause one to confuse this entity with bacterial endocarditis.

Reiter's syndrome is frequently chronic and may occasionally be differentiated from suspected gonococcal arthritis only after its chronicity becomes apparent when the patient fails to respond in the typical fashion to antibiotic therapy. Although the etiology of Reiter's syndrome remains unclear, the onset of Reiter's syndrome has been associated with a great variety of urogenital (Chlamydia and Ureaplasma) and enteric (Salmonella, Shigella, Yersinia, Campylobacter) pathogens. HLA tissue typing of leukocytes is useful in identifying the subgroup of patients in which Reiter's disease is most likely to develop. A disparate group of infections which are possibly related to Reiter's phenomenon has been associated with the entity of *reactive arthritis*. This process is a sterile inflammatory synovitis that follows infection with bacterial, viral, spirochetal, mycobacterial and parasitic agents. The most common examples are streptococci (group A and G), *Clostridium difficile*, staph toxic shock, Lyme disease, HIV, MTB and MAC, Giardia, Strongyloides and Cryptosporidium. The arthritis is asymmetric and additive, involving the lower extremities, especially the knees. Enthesopathy (pain at tendinous insertions) and dactylitis may be seen.

Bacterial Endocarditis

The patient with fever and polyarthritis may have bacterial endocarditis. The pathogenesis of the joint inflammation may be related either to direct bacterial invasion or to immunologic mechanisms. These patients will usually give a history of valvular heart disease and may show evidence of recent deterioration of their cardiovascular, renal, or neurologic status. Fever and weight loss may precede the presentation of the patients to the physician by weeks or even months. Other details of historical importance should include possible precipitating invasive procedures such as dental manipulation or GU tract surgery. The physical examination may lead to further suspicion of endocarditis if evidence of embolic or immunologic events are found, such as petechiae, Roth spots, splenomegaly, or microscopic hematuria. Clinical evidence of new or increased aortic or mitral regurgitation is a very important finding. On rare occasions a patient will have symptoms and signs of bacterial endocarditis with negative blood cultures. In such a patient, atrial myxoma and marantic endocarditis must be considered, in addition to culture-negative infective endocarditis.

Acute Rheumatic Fever

The combination of a murmur, fever, and polyarthritis may also suggest acute rheumatic fever. Occasionally the presence of subcutaneous nodules, chorea, or erythema marginatum will help support this latter diagnosis, but these manifestations are rare. The arthritis is frequently nonsymmetrical and involves the large joints; typically it is migratory, with new joints becoming involved within hours to days. The pain responds dramatically to aspirin. Rheumatic fever characteristically afflicts children more frequently than adults, occurring two to six weeks following a streptococcal pharyngitis, although the initial infection may not have been clinically evident. Recurrent bouts are not uncommon.

Infectious Hepatitis

Another illness that may present with polyarthritis is infectious hepatitis in its early prodromal phase. These patients are usually not jaundiced when the arthritis is present and may show only such nonspecific findings as fever, nausea, vomiting, and lassitude. Many hepatitis victims are young, and clues to this diagnosis include recent travel to an area of high endemicity, exposure of the patient to others with known "yellow jaundice," sharing of needles for illicit drug use, or close personal contact in situations of poor sanitation, as in homes for the mentally retarded.

The liver is generally quite tender on percussion or palpation, and splenomegaly may be found. Frequently in the early phase of hepatitis, the peripheral WBC count is low, with a relative increase in lymphocytes and some atypical lymphocytes as well. Thus in a patient with unsuspected early hepatitis, the finding of polyarthritis, leukopenia, splenomegaly, and fever may suggest the diagnosis of SLE or another collagen vascular disease. Pain over the liver on percussion or palpation and serologic investigation for hepatitis viruses may help distinguish this illness from classical lupus. Although the arthritis syndrome may be seen with any form of hepatitis, it is usually seen in the type B variety.

Parvovirus

The cause of childhood's fifth disease (erythema infectiosum) can infect adults also. When it does, a symmetric small joint polyarthritis often develops, with morning stiffness reminiscent of rheumatoid arthritis. Some patients have a macular or erythematous eruption with subsequent desquamation. Most victims of this arthritis are women.

Rubella and Mumps Arthritis

At times extensive workups for polyarthritis overlook the simple history of exposure of the patient to rubella or rubella vaccine. The classic rash of rubella is faint, maculopapular, pink, and blanching, and begins on the face and neck. Fine petechiae on the palate and enlarged lymph nodes in the suboccipital and postauricular area are usually present. Occasionally thrombocytopenia is noted. The arthritis in this disease is usually self limited.

History is also crucial in the diagnosis of mumps polyarthritis, because the joint inflammation almost always begins one to two weeks after the parotitis has disappeared.

HIV Infection

Infection with HIV virus may be associated with a polyarthritis that is mediated by CD8 lymphocytes and thus associated in many patients with HLA-B27 positivity. This arthritis is severe and chronic, causing deformities in an asymmetric oligoarthritic pattern. A more mild arthritis is also seen in HIV patients not associated with HLA-B27.

Coccidioidomycosis

A fungal infection commonly associated with arthritis is coccidioidomycosis. This disease is usually associated with a respiratory illness, and in its primary form may resemble influenza with fever, chills, cough, and patchy lung infiltrates. At this stage, erythema nodosum and joint pains (probably an immunologic phenomenon) may be present. A coccidioidin skin test is usually positive at this time. This disease should be suspected in patients living or recently returning from the arid southwestern United States, from California to Texas. Careful epidemiologic history is very important, since patients may be exposed to coccidioidomycotic arthrospores in nonendemic regions, for example, by exposure to raw materials shipped from the Southwest to other areas of the country.

In most instances the disease is self limited. Rarely, however, progression or dissemination may supervene. If dissemination occurs, a chronic polyarthritis commonly is seen, and organisms may be found in the joint fluid and synovia. Dissemination of coccidioidomycosis is usually accompanied by conversion of the skin test from positive to negative, a persistently high antibody titer, and a sedimentation rate that fails to fall after the initial illness.

Sarcoidosis

Sarcoidosis must be considered when a patient presents with erythema nodosum and polyarthritis. Joint involvement is transient and symmetrical, involving the large joints and appearing at the onset of the disease; it is often accompanied by fever, erythema nodosum and bilateral hilar lymphadenopathy (Lofgren's syndrome). This presentation is seen most often in young women of Swedish, Irish and Puerto Rican descent (although it may be seen in other groups) and carries a good prognosis. Helpful diagnostic points are the absence of erythema over afflicted joints and the good response of the arthritis to colchicine, but not to aspirin. Erythema nodosum may also be seen in association with sulfonamide or other drug hypersensitivity, as well as with numerous other infectious disease processes. A destructive chronic form of arthritis occurs in sarcoidosis but is rare. The etiology of sarcoidosis remains unknown.

Arbovirus Arthritis

Just as a geographic history is important in considering coccidioidomycosis, it plays a crucial role in the diagnosis of the arbovirus infections, chikungunya and O'nyong-nyong fever. These illnesses are seen in Africa and Southeast Asia and may be imported to other countries by travelers to these regions. Fever, headache, and rash often accompany the arthritis, which is severe. In fact, chikungunya means "doubled-up" and describes the suffering of its victims. Other related alphaviruses may cause similar illnesses, e.g., Ross River, Mayaro, Sindbis and Ockelbo.

Rat-Bite Fever

Another form of infectious arthritis that is quite rare but should be considered in patients with fever, rash, and joint symptoms is rat-bite fever. This disease may be produced by either *Spirillum minus* or *Streptobacillus moniliformis*. The Spirillum infection occurs several weeks after the rat bite and may pursue a relapsing course. It is associated with an inflammatory response at the bite site during the time of acute illness, and a false-positive VDRL is present in 50 percent of cases. In the Streptobacillus infection, which is more commonly associated with arthritis, the incubation period is usually less than 10 days, although the resultant illness may be indistinguishable from that caused by *S. minus*. Occasionally Streptobacillus is spread by contaminated food, in which case the disease has sometimes been called Haverhill fever. Laboratory workers are at particular risk for infection with *S. moniliformis*.

Syphilitic Arthritis

In secondary syphilis, a polyarthritis is accompanied by fever, adenopathy, rash, and mucous membrane lesions. Syphilitic arthritis also occurs in the tertiary stage as manifested by neuropathic (Charcot's) or gummatous joints, or in congenital syphilis as recurrent hydrarthrosis (Clutton's joints).

Lyme Disease

Lyme disease is caused by *B. burgdorferi*, spread to humans via a tick bite. After an initial illness characterized by a flu-like syndrome and erythema at the bite site (erythema chronicum migrans), patients may develop chronic neurologic, cardiac or arthritic sequelae. Chronic arthritis may occur as early as two weeks or as late as two years after the initial illness. Patients develop recurring attacks of asymmetric large joint inflammation (especially the knee). Some develop Baker's cysts, and a small percent develop chronic rheumatoid-like inflammation, with pannus formation and erosion of bone and cartilage.

Lymphogranuloma Venereum Arthritis

In LGV, bilateral multilocular suppurative inguinal adenopathy is usually evident, the genital papule having gone unnoticed. The nodes can rupture, forming multiple draining sinuses and, in the female, rectal strictures. A careful search for present or recent clinical manifestations of LGV will usually help identify LGV as the cause of the polyarthritis. Serology may be helpful.

Whipple's Disease

In Whipple's disease, the polyarthritis may antedate by years the other manifestations of this disorder, which include abdominal pain and diarrhea with malabsorption, steatorrhea, hyperpigmentation, and lymphadenopathy. The diagnosis of this entity is suggested by the presence of large numbers of PAS-positive macrophages on small bowel biopsy; if available, electron microscopy may show bacillary organisms in small bowel mucosa and lymph nodes, and the polymerase chain reaction (PCR) may identify the presence of the causative organism, *Tropheryma whippeli*. After antibiotic therapy the GI symptoms are markedly alleviated and the above-mentioned bacilli disappear.

In addition to acute rheumatic fever and sarcoidosis, mentioned above, there are other noninfectious polyarthritis syndromes that may simulate infection. These are listed in Table 8.2.

TABLE 8.2. NONINFECTIOUS POLYARTHRITIS

Collagen-vascular disease,[a] especially SLE, rheumatoid arthritis, juvenile rheumatoid arthritis
Neoplasms: leukemia, lymphoma, rarely others
Sarcoidosis
Inflammatory bowel disease
Metabolic: gout,[a] pseudogout,[a] achronosis
Serum sickness
Hemoglobinopathies
Psoriasis
Hypo-, hypergammaglobulinemia
Amyloidosis
S/P intestinal bypass for obesity
Behcet's syndrome
Familial Mediterranean fever
Palindromic rheumatism

[a] Most common causes.

TABLE 8.3. DIAGNOSTIC CHART: INFECTIOUS POLYARTHRITIS—SELECTED ETIOLOGIES

Disease	Etiology, Epidemiology, and/or Pathogenesis	Clinical Signs	Diagnosis[b]	Initial Therapy (Alternative Rx in Parentheses)
A. Bacterial infections[a]				
1. Disseminated gonococcal infection	Venereal spread. Focus from which bacteremia occurs may be genital, rectal, or pharyngeal.	Fever and leukocytosis may be present or absent. Patient not extremely toxic. Early polyarthritis frequently progresses to involvement of 1 or 2 joints only. Petechiae, papules, or vesicles are common, usually on distal extremities around infected joints. They are typically few in number. Tenosynovitis, especially of wrist or ankle, is characteristic.	Smear and culture of joint fluid, petechiae, and (in males) urethral exudate. Culture of blood, joint fluid, cervix, rectum, urethra, pharynx. Joint fluid: Group III[b].	Ceftriaxone (ciprofloxacin).

2. Meningococcemia	Disease disseminates in community from the asymptomatic nasopharyngeal carrier. Meningitis results from bacteremic spread from nasopharynx.	Illness may progress rapidly, with fever, shock, petechiae, ecchymoses and DIC. WBCs may be extremely high (30–40,000), but may also be normal or low. Illness is less fulminant in some cases in which meningitis predominates. Occasionally the rare syndrome of chronic meningococcemia with arthralgias or arthritis is noted.	Smear and culture of joint fluid and skin lesions. Blood cultures. Gram stain of buffy coat. CSF studies may show evidence of meningitis. Joint fluid: Group III.[b]	Penicillin G, (3rd generation cephalosporins).

(continued)

TABLE 8.3. (continued) DIAGNOSTIC CHART: INFECTIOUS POLYARTHRITIS—SELECTED ETIOLOGIES

Disease	Etiology, Epidemiology, and/or Pathogenesis	Clinical Signs	Diagnosis[b]	Initial Therapy (Alternative Rx in Parentheses)
3. Subacute bacterial endocarditis	Usually occurs in setting of preexisting rheumatic, arteriosclerotic, or congenital heart disease, or with prosthetic valves, idiopathic hypertrophic subaortic stenosis, or mitral valve prolapse.	Fever generally present and may be associated with polyarthralgias or polyarthritis, monoarthritis, back pain, petechiae, anemia, hematuria, and/or deterioration in cardiac, renal or neurologic status.	Blood cultures are positive in 85% if 5 separate specimens are drawn; more than 5 have small additional yield. Positive rheumatoid factor in 50% of patients who have had disease longer than 6 weeks. Low serum complement if nephritis present. An elevated ESR is a common lab abnormality. Gram stain and culture emboli if an embolectomy is performed. If blood cultures are negative, perform fungal and Q fever serologies; inoculate small amounts of blood	If therapy must be instituted before cultures and sensitivities known: Ampicillin + gentamicin (vancomycin + gentamicin). Prosthetic valve: vancomycin + gentamicin ± rifampin.

			into culture medium to dilute serum antibody; do buffy coat smear, stain ear lobe histocytes, culture for cell-wall deficient organisms, and discuss with the microbiologist any additional media or cultural techniques that could be attempted. Cultures should be held for 3 wks. Echocardiography is helpful in documenting complications but is of less value in establishing or excluding the diagnosis. Joint fluid is not diagnostic.	
4. Rat-bite fever (S. moniliformis)	Rat bite or ingestion of contaminated food.	Fever, polyarthritis, maculopapular or petechial rash on extremities, especially around joints.	Culture of blood, wound, joint fluid. Serology.	Penicillin G, tetracycline.

(continued)

TABLE 8.3. (continued) DIAGNOSTIC CHART: INFECTIOUS POLYARTHRITIS—SELECTED ETIOLOGIES

Disease	Etiology, Epidemiology, and/or Pathogenesis	Clinical Signs	Diagnosis[b]	Initial Therapy (Alternative Rx in Parentheses)
B. Viral infections				
1. Mumps	Respiratory spread by infected patient.	Fever, parotitis, pancreatitis, encephalitis, orchitis; arthritis usually follows parotitis by 1–2 weeks.	WBC normal or low. Amylase may be elevated. Serology helpful. Other viral diseases may simulate mumps, especially enteroviral infection. Joint fluid Group II.[b]	Symptomatic.
2. Rubella	Polyarthritis syndrome may appear after rubella vaccination or natural rubella infection in young adults, especially women. Airborne spread from infected patients.	Fever, pink macular rash, adenopathy (especially postauricular and occipital) are the clinical findings. The joint discomfort may persist for weeks after the rash and fever have disappeared. WBC may be normal or low.	Serology; recovery of virus from nasopharyngeal washings. Joint fluid Group II.[b]	No specific therapy.

3. Hepatitis (especially with hepatitis B)	Parenteral or nonparenteral spread from infected individuals.	Symmetric, migratory polyarthritis of small and large joints and urticaria may be part of prodrome. Tender enlarged liver, anorexia, jaundice, elevated SGOT, low or normal WBC with atypical lymphocytosis, low or normal ESR.	Serology. Most arthritis seen in hepatitis B. During polyarthritis, see low serum complement and presence of Hb_sAg with low complement in joint fluid. Liver biopsy characteristic. Gp I or II joint fluid.[b]	No specific therapy.
4. Parvovirus	Respiratory spread.	Fever, rash, small joints of hands and knees. Symmetric polyarthritis. May have morning stiffness. Rash may desquamate. Illness may be biphasic with rash and arthritis following flu-like illness in 1–2 weeks.	Serology. Joint fluid Group I or II.[b]	No specific therapy.
5. HIV infection	Inoculation of body fluids.	May see a mild polyarthritis or a severe chronic pauciarticular form that causes permanent deformities.	Serology. Joint fluid Group I or II.[b]	No specific therapy.

(continued)

TABLE 8.3. (continued) DIAGNOSTIC CHART: INFECTIOUS POLYARTHRITIS—SELECTED ETIOLOGIES

Disease	Etiology, Epidemiology, and/or Pathogenesis	Clinical Signs	Diagnosis[b]	Initial Therapy (Alternative Rx in Parentheses)
C. Fungal infections: coccidioidomycosis	In US, seen in patients living in arid Southwest or in those exposed to athrospores by products transported from endemic to nonendemic regions.	Initial exposure usually a transient self-limited illness, suggesting URI but may have arthralgias, erythema nodosum, eosinophilia, and high ESR. May progress to chronic arthritis.	In primary infection, culture of sputum, serology, and skin test helpful. Smears and cultures of sputum and joint fluid as well as synovial biopsy should be done in disseminated disease. Serology and skin tests helpful.	Uncomplicated primary form: no specific therapy. Progressive or disseminated form: amphotericin B (itraconazole).
D. Spirochetal infections				
1. Secondary syphilis	Venereal spread.	Fever, lymphadenopathy, maculopapular rash, especially on palms and soles, occurring 2 weeks to 6 months after chancre, occasionally associated with polyarthralgia or polyarthritis.	Dark-field of moist lesions; serology. Joint fluid is not diagnostic.	Penicillin (doxycycline).

2. Rat-bite fever (*Spirillum minus*)	Rat bite.	Fever; bite site flares when acute illness begins. Maculopapular rash on abdomen extending to extremities and becoming petechial. May involve palms and soles. Joint involvement is less common in this form of rat bite fever than in the streptobacillus infection described previously.	Inoculate blood or wound aspirate into mice or guinea pigs. Dark field of bite, rash, blood, or node aspirate. Serology. False-positive VDRL frequent.	Penicillin G, doxycycline.
3. Lyme Disease	Tick bite (usually unnoticed).	Erythema chronicum migrans at bite site (spreading red lesion with central clearing). Then flu-like illness with subsequent neurologic, cardiac or oligoarticular arthritic phenomena. Joints involved are large, usually the knee, asymmetric, with occasional Baker's cyst formation and occasional development of rheumatoid arthritis-like picture.	Serology. PCR has detected DNA sequences in blood, CSF, skin, urine and synovial fluid.	Ceftriaxone (doxycycline).

(continued)

TABLE 8.3. (continued) DIAGNOSTIC CHART: INFECTIOUS POLYARTHRITIS—SELECTED ETIOLOGIES

Disease	Etiology, Epidemiology, and/or Pathogenesis	Clinical Signs	Diagnosis[b]	Initial Therapy (Alternative Rx in Parentheses)
E. Chlamydial infections: LGV	Venereal spread.	Primary evanescent painless genital papule-vesicle, followed in 30 days by inguinal adenopathy. Rectal disease with diarrhea may be seen in females and homosexual males. LGV may be accompanied by polyarthralgias, polyarthritis, and myalgias.	Serologic test helpful. Although lymph-node biopsy shows characteristic pathology, in general this procedure is not performed, since fistula formation is a complication.	Doxycycline.

F. Miscellaneous processes			
1. Whipple's disease	Bacterium: Tropheryma whippeli. Seen primarily in males.	Abdominal pain, malabsorption, diarrhea, polyarthritis; CNS and ophthalmologic complications occasionally seen. Joint symptoms may precede GI symptoms by years.	Biopsy of small bowel, lymph node, rectum, with special stains. Electron microscopy may show bacterial forms in small bowel lamina propria. PCR may identify the pathogen.	Doxycycline.
2. Reiter's disease	Appears to be sexually transmitted and may be seen with change in sexual partner. Chlamydia may be important as etiologic precipitant. At times follows diarrheal illness, especially Shigella or Yersinia infection. Seen primarily in males with HLA type W27.	Arthritis, conjunctivitis, urethritis, and skin lesions (mucosal ulcerations and keratoderma blenorrhagica) make up the classical tetrad, but many patients have only one or two of the manifestations. Course may be relapsing. No dramatic response to any therapy.	Calcaneal spurs on heel x-ray. Sacroiliitis on pelvic x-ray. Joint fluid Gp II;[b] complement elevated. HLA typing may help identify patients in whom Reiter's disease is most likely to be seen.	No specific therapy.

(continued)

TABLE 8.3. *(continued)* DIAGNOSTIC CHART: INFECTIOUS POLYARTHRITIS—SELECTED ETIOLOGIES

Disease	Etiology, Epidemiology, and/or Pathogenesis	Clinical Signs	Diagnosis[b]	Initial Therapy (Alternative Rx in Parentheses)
3. Acute rheumatic fever	Late nonsuppurative complication of Group A streptococcal pharyngitis.	Fever, migratory asymmetric polyarthritis, erythema marginatum, subcutaneous nodules, chorea, and carditis (involvement of pericardium, myocardium, or endocardium) may be seen. Usually a disease of children. Frequently misdiagnosed initially in adults. The arthritis does not last longer than 3 weeks; if it does, a different diagnosis should be entertained.	Clinical criteria are important. Streptococcal serology helpful. Joint fluid: Group II.[b] Dramatic response of joint pains to aspirin in high doses. EKG may show evidence of pericarditis or myocarditis.	Aspirin. Corticosteroids for severe carditis.
4. SLE	Etiology unknown; seen primarily in young women.	Fever, polyarthritis, nephritis, anemia, leukopenia,	Elevated ESR. Antinuclear antibody positive in 95%. Anti-DNA antibody in	Aspirin, corticosteroids, immunosuppressive

POLYARTHRITIS

5. Serum sickness	Reaction to heterologous serum administration, drugs, or insect bites. May occur as part of a response to an infectious agent. Related to antigen excess states.	Fever, polyarthritis, nephritis, urticaria, other allergic phenomena, neuritis.	ESR may be normal or increased. Eosinophilia. Decreased serum complement. Joint fluid: Group I or II.[b]	Symptomatic. Corticosteroids are helpful.
6. Sarcoidosis	Etiology unknown. In US, blacks are affected more frequently than whites. Disease especially in southeastern U.S.	Pulmonary infiltrates, polyarthritis, adenopathy, skin lesions, iritis, hypercalcemia, heart block.	Biopsy of lymph node, lung, skin, liver, conjunctiva; Kveim skin test may be helpful if good antigen available. Skin test anergy in many. Joint fluid: Group I.[b]	Arthritis may respond to colchicine, but does not respond well to aspirin. Corticosteroids may be indicated for serious disease involving the eye, myocardium, CNS or lungs.

(Previous row continuation: thrombocytopenia, splenomegaly, polyserositis, and other evidence of vasculitis may be present either singly or in various combinations. 60%. Chronic biologic false-positive VDRL in 15%. Joint fluid: Group I or II.[b] agents.)

(continued)

TABLE 8.3. (continued) DIAGNOSTIC CHART: INFECTIOUS POLYARTHRITIS—SELECTED ETIOLOGIES

Disease	Etiology, Epidemiology, and/or Pathogenesis	Clinical Signs	Diagnosis[b]	Initial Therapy (Alternative Rx in Parentheses)
7. Rheumatoid arthritis	Etiology unknown. Female preponderance. Average age of onset is third or fourth decade; 2–3% of adult population in U.S. may be affected.	A generalized systemic disease associated with polyarthritis. Symmetrical involvement of multiple joints with periarticular swelling and morning stiffness. May be relapsing or progressive and cause severe deformity. Also see muscular atrophy, subcutaneous nodules.	Fever, malaise, anemia, positive ANA, positive rheumatoid factor in serum and synovial fluid. X-rays characteristic, as are synovial fluid and biopsy of synovium or subcutaneous nodule. Synovial fluid complement may be decreased, especially if rheumatoid factor present in joint fluid. Joint fluid: Group II.[b]	Symptomatic; anti-inflammatory agents, chloroquine, gold, cytotoxic agents.
8. Juvenile rheumatoid arthritis	Etiology unknown. Most cases in children but can occur in young adults, especially males.	Begins before puberty in most. More likely than rheumatoid arthritis to cause marked fever, rash, and iritis. Growth and developmental abnormalities may occur.	Rheumatoid factor usually not present. X-rays and synovial biopsy characteristic. Joint fluid: Group II.[b]	Symptomatic; anti-inflammatory agents.

Cervical involvement common (50%). In young adults with variant of this disease, prolonged hectic fever with high ESR and transient rash may occur for weeks to months prior to joint symptoms, causing difficulty in diagnosis.

	WNL	Non-Inflammatory Group 1	Inflammatory Group II	Purulent Group III
WBC/mm^3	<50	<3000	3000–50,000	50,000–300,000
% PMN	<25	<25	>70	>90
Volume (ml)	<4	>4	>4	>4
Color	Clear/yellow	Yellow	Yellow-white	White
Clarity	Transparent	Transparent	Transparent-opaque	Opaque
Viscosity	Good	Fair	Poor	Very poor
Glucose	= serum	= serum	= serum	<50% of serum glucose

[a] Bacteremia with any organism may produce monoarthritis or polyarthritis, but the organisms shown should be especially considered.
[b] Joint Fluid Types (Data regarding joint fluid types are supplied when available.)

Adapted from McCarty, Lea & Febiger, ed #12 p. 65.

9

JAUNDICE

The clinical finding of jaundice always indicates a pathologic state. Its causes are numerous, but the common denominator is hyperbilirubinemia, the accumulation of bile pigments in the blood. Such accumulation may be prehepatic, hepatic, or posthepatic in origin, resulting from excess pigment production, defective processing by the liver, or obstruction of the excretion of bile in the biliary tract, respectively. When the serum level of bilirubin reaches 2.5 mg %, yellow staining of tissues is evident, and this is most easily detectable in areas of the body where structures have large components of elastic tissue, e.g., the conjunctivae, the palate, and the sublingual mucosa.

Before discussing the specific infections that cause jaundice, it should be noted that in a patient with underlying liver disease, jaundice may also appear or worsen from a variety of nonspecific causes. For example, a patient with cirrhosis may show deterioration of his liver function when distant infection supervenes. Another possible point of confusion in evaluating an infected patient with jaundice is the possibility that the drugs being used to treat the patient might be responsible for causing jaundice. Anti-infective agents may cause (a) hemolysis (e.g., nitrofurantoin, para-aminosalicylic acid (PAS), sulfonamides, penicillin, cephalothin,

TABLE 9.1. JAUNDICE

A. Hemolysis associated with infection
  1. Malaria
  2. Babesiosis
  3. *C. perfringens* toxemia
  4. Bartonellosis
  5. Infection in patients with abnormal RBCs

B. Extrahepatic obstruction associated with infection
  1. Cholangitis
     a. Secondary to common duct stone
     b. Secondary to pancreatic disease
     c. Secondary to cholecystitis
     d. Secondary to carcinoma of ampulla of vater
  2. May be simulated by drug toxicity (e.g., erythromycin)
  3. May be simulated by gonococcal perihepatitis, infectious hepatitis, or alcoholic hepatitis

C. Hepatic injury associated with infection
  1. Specific infections
     a. Gonococcal perihepatitis
     b. Viral hepatitis
     c. Infectious mononucleosis
     d. Leptospirosis
     e. Syphilis
     f. Q fever
     g. Neonates: herpes simplex, rubella, CMV infection
     h. Outside U.S.: yellow fever, clonorchiasis, ascariasis, schistosomiasis
     i. Rarely: borreliosis, congenital or secondary syphilis, coxsackie infection, psittacosis, CMV infection
  2. Bloodstream infections
     a. bacteremia (arterial)
     b. pylephlebitis
  3. Liver abscess
     a. pyogenic
     b. amebic

quinine, isoniazid), (b) direct liver injury (isoniazid, PAS, rifampin, sulfonamides, dilantin, tetracycline), and (c) cholestasis, indistinguishable from hepatic obstruction (e.g., erythromycin estolate). Any number of drugs are capable of producing jaundice and fever, and in a patient with this symptom complex, an adverse drug reaction must be considered.

Jaundice associated with infection may be prehepatic, hepatic, or posthepatic (obstructive) (Table 9.1). In infection the most important prehepatic cause is hemolysis. Hepatic causes of jaundice result from direct liver injury in a variety of infectious diseases and probably represent the most common mechanisms of jaundice associated with infection. Obstructive jaundice associated with infection is usually related to diseases of the pancreas or biliary tract.

INFECTIONS ASSOCIATED WITH HEMOLYSIS

Dramatic hemolysis productive of jaundice is seen with relatively few disorders and is suggested by a falling hematocrit, increased reticulocyte count, increased serum lactic dehydrogenase, elevated levels of plasma hemoglobin, and a falling haptoglobin, with a peripheral blood smear that demonstrates schistocytes or microspherocytes. The bilirubin is mostly unconjugated and is therefore absent from the urine. Except in neonates, bilirubin levels due to hemolysis alone are rarely greater than 5 mg %, and, if they are, hepatic dysfunction is likely.

Malaria is usually suspected in the syndrome of fever, rigors, and hemolysis, especially in patients who have had exposure to an endemic area or to contaminated blood or needles. Examination of the peripheral blood smear will almost always readily demonstrate the parasite.

Babesiosis resembles malaria clinically and also is caused by an intraerythrocytic parasite. It is spread by ticks and is endemic in several islands off the New England coast.

C. perfringens septicemia, seen particularly in postabortal or puerperal states, may produce rapid and extreme hemolysis because of the alpha toxin produced by the organism. Microspherocytes are especially common in the peripheral smear of patients with clostridial toxemia. With other *C. perfringens* infections such as gangrene, significant hemolysis occurs much more rarely.

Mycoplasma infection may be associated with significant hemolysis during convalescence. Syphilis and other agents, particularly viruses, may cause paroxysmal cold hemoglobinuria. Bartonellosis typically produces fever and hemolysis, but this disorder is localized to the Andes region of South America, and lack of travel to that area effectively rules out this diagnosis. Many other infections may be accompanied by hemolytic episodes, but except for those mentioned above, the hemolysis is usually overshadowed by the clinical syndrome of the infection producing it—typhoid fever or bacterial endocarditis, for example.

Finally, patients with abnormal RBCs or chronic low-grade hemolysis may have significant hemolytic episodes triggered by an acute infection. For example, this is seen in patients with sickle cell anemia, G–6–PD deficiency, or paroxysmal nocturnal hemoglobinuria (PNH). (See also Chapter 14, *Hematologic Changes Associated with Infection*).

INFECTIONS ASSOCIATED WITH POSTHEPATIC JAUNDICE

Posthepatic jaundice is caused by obstruction of the biliary tract that is complicated by an infection behind the obstruction. Such obstruction results most frequently from stones in the common duct or from tumor, but stricture of the common duct, pancreatitis, and cholecystitis may also be responsible.

Fever, chills, right upper quadrant pain, and jaundice suggest the possibility of ascending cholangitis, an infection associated with extrahepatic biliary obstruction. The liver function tests will show elevation of direct-reacting bilirubin and alkaline phosphatase with only minimally elevated transaminases. The WBC count is frequently elevated. Blood cultures should be drawn, since they may detect an associated bacteremia. The obstruction must be relieved surgically. In some patients, episodes of relapsing fever and chills occur, which have been termed Charcot's biliary fever.

There are a number of other intraabdominal processes that may resemble cholangitis. Cholecystitis may present with fever and pain in the right upper quadrant or midepigastrium, and 20 percent of patients may be jaundiced because of either an associated common duct stone or edema of the biliary ducts associated with the gallbladder inflammation. Pancreatitis may cause fever and midepigastric pain, and an edematous pancreas may obstruct biliary outflow.

Diagnosis of these obstructive disorders in the jaundiced patient is usually made by sonography or CT scans. It should be remembered that an obstructed common duct may not dilate for several days. Also, it is a common misconception that an obstructed cystic duct results in an enlarged gallbladder. If chronic cholelithiasis is present, a stone impacted in the cystic duct will not expand a chronically scarred gallbladder. On the other hand, sudden cystic duct obstruction in the presence of a normal gallbladder, for example due to malignancy, may cause the gallbladder to expand. Occasionally x-rays of the abdomen reveal stones in the right upper quadrant or air in the biliary tree that has been produced by gas-forming bacteria. However, it should be stressed that emergency decompression is indicated in any patient in whom extrahepatic biliary obstruction with secondary infection is strongly suspected. At times, transduodenal or transhepatic cannulation of bile ducts can relieve obstruction of main bile ducts or of the common duct. Also, a sick patient with cystic duct obstruction may be drained (temporarily) by cholecystostomy.

Occasionally intrahepatic obstruction simulates surgically-correctable jaundice. Infectious hepatitis, which will be discussed later, may present an obstructive picture with minimally elevated transaminases and extreme elevations in alkaline phosphatase and bilirubin. However, although viral hepatitis A or B may begin with fever and chills, the patient usually becomes afebrile when jaundice is evident. Alcoholic hepatitis often presents an obstructive pattern of blood chemistries, along with fever, right upper quadrant pain, and at times, significant leukocytosis.

An unusual syndrome that mimics cholangitis is gonococcal perihepatitis or the "Fitzhugh-Curtis syndrome." In women with gonococcal pelvic inflammatory disease, the infection can spread to the upper abdomen and cause a fibrinous peritonitis over the liver, producing right upper quadrant pain, fever, a hepatic friction rub, and, occasionally, jaundice. Interestingly, the gall bladder may not visualize in this condition, but this abnormality and the associated symptomatology will remit with antigonococcal therapy.

INFECTIONS ASSOCIATED WITH HEPATIC JAUNDICE

Infectious hepatitis is now known to result from infection with one of at least five, and possibly more, antigenically distinct viruses. These are currently designated as hepatitis viruses A, B, C, D and E. Patients may have prodromal symptoms of anorexia, nausea or vomiting, polyarthritis, urticaria, and rarely, fever and chills. When the jaundice begins and the diagnosis becomes apparent, the fever usually returns toward normal and the liver is often enlarged and tender. Splenomegaly may sometimes be seen. The WBC count is normal or low, and atypical lymphocytes may be present in large numbers. The laboratory evaluation is helpful in hepatitis because the SGOT and SGPT levels are usually greater than 400 units; the bilirubin and alkaline phosphatase levels are extremely variable. A helpful determination is the sedimentation rate, which is frequently normal or low.

Hepatitis may be produced by other organisms that are not "hepatitis viruses." For example, EB virus mononucleosis may produce hepatic injury clinically indistinguishable from that seen in infection due to the hepatitis viruses. However, patients with infectious mononucleosis will usually show more marked involvement of the lymph nodes, spleen, pharynx, and peripheral blood. Infectious mononucleosis is usually readily diagnosed serologically. Other acute infections may resemble EB virus mono and are said to cause the "mono syndrome" e.g., CMV, toxoplasma, HHV-6, rubella, acute HIV and herpes simplex. These may all produce hepatic inflammation. Similarly, leptospirosis produces a nonspecific hepatitis. This disease is often accompanied by high fevers and shaking chills, myalgias, conjunctivitis, aseptic meningitis, renal damage, and neutrophilia. However, it should be remembered that most patients with leptospirosis are not jaundiced. Secondary syphilis may be complicated by hepatitis, especially in homosexual males. A clue to a syphilitic etiology is the disproportionate elevation in alkaline phosphate and bilirubin compared with transaminases.

Finally, up to one-third of patients with Q fever may have hepatitis and jaundice. Though these patients usually present with prominent headache and pneumonitis, these symptoms are not always found. Q fever is notable among the rickettsial diseases for its lack of a rash and the negative Weil-Felix reaction. A history of contact with livestock, especially cattle, may be a helpful clue. It is one of the causes of a granulomatous hepatitis.

In neonates, jaundice may result from specific infection with herpes simplex, rubella, and CMV infection. Outside the United States, parasitic infections, especially clonorchiasis, ascariasis, and schistosomiasis, are frequently important causes of jaundice. Although amebiasis may cause severe liver involvement, jaundice is rarely seen. Many other agents are capable of causing hepatitis and jaundice.

Bacteremia of many diverse etiologies may be associated with jaundice that results not only from hemolysis, but also from direct liver injury *per se*. This phenomenon has been observed particularly in sepsis or severe infection with *Streptococcus pneumoniae* and other streptococci, *K. pneumoniae*, *S. typhi* and other salmonellae, *Bacteroides fragilis* and *E. coli*. Liver biopsy in these instances may reveal small focal collections of PMLs. Associated with septicemia, this hepatic lesion usually remits when the bloodstream infection is controlled, but occasionally may progress to actual macroabscess formation.

With intraabdominal suppurative processes such as appendicitis or diverticulitis, mesenteric and portal vein bacteremia may occur, producing a pylephlebitis. In this syndrome, patients may be severely ill and have chills, fever, right upper quadrant pain, and liver enlargement, as well as jaundice.

Another cause of jaundice produced by disease within the liver is hepatic abscess. This entity is usually pyogenic in origin and occurs most commonly with extrahepatic biliary tract obstruction or intraabdominal suppurations. Liver abscess may follow abdominal trauma, bacteremia, tumor necrosis with subsequent infection or may be entirely cryptogenic.

The so-called classic syndrome of pyogenic abscess (chills, fever, right upper quadrant pain, tenderness, and jaundice) is not seen in all cases. Many of these patients are not acutely ill and present with FUO or nonspecific constitutional complaints. Abnormal sonogram or CT scan and chest x-rays demonstrating an elevated or paralyzed hemidiaphragm with atelectasis or pleural effusions are common. Mild jaundice and elevated alkaline phosphatase are frequent findings. Occasionally abdominal x-rays reveal an air fluid level within the liver. The most common causative organisms are the enteric aerobic Gram-negative rods and anaerobic bacteria. Aerobic Gram-positive cocci are also important causes of liver abscess, especially in children with septicemia.

Amebic liver abscess usually resembles pyogenic abscess clinically, but a few differences have been noted. Amebic abscesses tend to be single and larger. Patients with amebic disease are usually less acutely ill, and jaundice is less frequent. Distinguishing between amebic and pyogenic abscesses is difficult, because patients with amebic abscess only rarely have overt evidence of GI symptoms and only rarely demonstrate trophozoites in the stool. Eosinophilia is not a characteristic finding in amebic disease. One helpful clue is that if an amebic abscess is aspirated, the foul odor characteristic of anaerobic pyogenic infection is not found.

The diagnostic armamentarium is the same as for pyogenic abscess, with the important addition of amebic serology, which is positive in close to 100% of cases of amebic liver abscess. Also, a clinical trial of dihydroemetine or chloroquine frequently results in improvement (a clinical trial of metronidazole may cause improvement in either amebic or anaerobic pyogenic abscess, and thus is not useful as a diagnostic tool). Aspiration of a suspected abscess may successfully distinguish between amebic and pyogenic origin. Absence of bacteria on Gram stain and culture with or without trophozoites suggests an amebic etiology, whereas the presence of bacteria proves a pyogenic cause. However, results of aspiration must be interpreted with caution. For example, trophozoites are unlikely to be seen unless the wall of the abscess is aspirated, and pyogenic organisms may be found in an amebic abscess that has been secondarily infected with bacteria. The distinction between pyogenic and amebic abscess is obviously important, since pyogenic abscess usually requires surgical drainage and specific antibiotics, whereas amebic abscess responds to antiamebic chemotherapy with or without needle aspiration. Surgical drainage is rarely indicated in amebic abscess except for lesions in the left lobe, which may rupture into the pericardium, and in abscesses that are rapidly expanding and threatening to rupture.

TABLE 9.2. DIAGNOSTIC CHART: JAUNDICE—SELECTED ETIOLOGIES

Disease	Etiology, Epidemiology, and/or Pathogenesis	Clinical Signs	Diagnosis	Initial Therapy (Alternative Rx in Parentheses)
A. Hemolytic jaundice: *C. perfringens* toxemia	Exotoxin formation in necrotic infected tissue. Seen primarily in obstetrical patients, especially with septic abortion. Seen only rarely with severe gas gangrene related to trauma or tumor necrosis.	Severe intravascular hemolysis associated with shock, renal failure, and fever. Rapid onset of jaundice.	Evidence of severe hemolysis (anemia, increased bilirubin, pink serum, dark urine). Measure plasma hemoglobin and haptoglobin. Reticulocyte count. Peripheral smear may show microspherocytes. X-rays of infected area may show gas formation in tissues. Obtain anaerobic blood cultures. Obtain necrotic tissue and Gram stain, looking for fat Gram-positive rods. Culture tissue anaerobically.	Surgical debridement. High-dose penicillin G. Hyperbaric oxygen is of debatable value. (Most clinicians do not use gas gangrene antitoxin.)
B. Extrahepatic obstruction 1. Pancreatitis	Gallstones and alcoholism are the most frequent conditions	Jaundice associated with fever, midepigastric pain frequently radiating to	Elevated direct bilirubin, alkaline phosphatase. High serum lipase + amylase.	Nothing by mouth. Nasogastric suction. Antibiotics usually

(continued)

TABLE 9.2. *(continued)* DIAGNOSTIC CHART: JAUNDICE-SELECTED ETIOLOGIES

Disease	Etiology, Epidemiology, and/or Pathogenesis	Clinical Signs	Diagnosis	Initial Therapy (Alternative Rx in Parentheses)
	associated with pancreatitis, but the exact pathogenesis is still obscure.	the back, associated with nausea and vomiting. May have peritoneal signs in severe cases along with abdominal hemorrhage and Grey-Turner's and Cullen's signs. Hypotension may be present.	WBCs may be elevated. Serum calcium frequently low in severe cases. A KUB may show gallstones, pancreatic calcifications, or a sentinel loop reflecting an inflamed pancreas.	not needed except for complications such as infected pseudocyst or abscess. Surgery may be indicated for complications or for correcting surgical causes of pancreatitis.
2. Cholecystitis	Primarily seen in middle-aged females.	Jaundice associated with intermittent colicky or continuous right upper quadrant pain radiating to the back and right shoulder and occasionally to the midepigastrium or even left side of abdomen. Frequently some fever, but occasionally high fever and chills, which may recur with intermittent biliary obstruction.	Elevation of direct bilirubin, alkaline phosphatase, and at times, WBCs. KUB may show stones in biliary system. Occasionally gas is noted in gall bladder or ducts if infection present. Sonography. CT scan. At times laparotomy may be required.	Surgery. Use of antibiotics controversial unless patient appears septic or obvious infection is noted at time of surgery.

3. Cholangitis	Generally secondary to obstruction of common duct, whether by stone, neoplasm, stricture, or pancreatitis.	Jaundice with hectic fever, chills with right upper quadrant pain and tenderness.	Direct bilirubin, alkaline phosphatase, and WBCs elevated. SGOT usually less than 200, but rarely may be as high as 1,000 units. X-rays: proceed diagnostically as for cholecystitis, but diagnosis must be made rapidly. Early laparotomy is indicated if diagnosis cannot be ruled out quickly by noninvasive means.	Surgery and antibiotics directed against anaerobes, streptococci, and Gram-negative bacilli (No single regimen is accepted by all, but a combination of ampicillin-sulbactam and gentamicin provides coverage against most pathogens associated with this entity.)
C. Hepatic injury 1. Caused by a specific infection a. Gonococcal perihepatitis (Fitzhugh-Curtis syndrome)	A rare but treatable complication of gonococcal pelvic infection.	History of pelvic inflammatory disease followed by fever, right upper quadrant and shoulder pain, and occasionally mild jaundice. A friction rub	Gonococci usually found on *cervical* culture. Should also culture rectum, blood, and pharynx.	Ceftriaxone (ciprofloxacin)

(continued)

TABLE 9.2. *(continued)* DIAGNOSTIC CHART: JAUNDICE-SELECTED ETIOLOGIES

Disease	Etiology, Epidemiology, and/or Pathogenesis	Clinical Signs	Diagnosis	Initial Therapy (Alternative Rx in Parentheses)
		may be heard over the liver. Hepatic tenderness noted on physical exam. Failure of gall bladder to visualize on cholecystogram is common and may be misleading.		
b. Viral hepatitis	At least five, and possibly more, types exist. Types A and E are usually spread by fecal-oral routes, hepatitis B and C by parenteral and sexual exposure, and delta is superimposed on chronic hepatitis B victims.	Hepatitis is associated with severe malaise, fever, anorexia, nausea, right upper quadrant pain and tenderness. These findings generally precede the jaundice by several days and some patients never become jaundiced. Hepatitis B is more likely to produce severe illness and at times presents with a serum sickness-like syndrome during the early phase of illness.	Liver function tests usually show very elevated SGOT and SGPT (>400 units), prolonged prothrombin time, variable alkaline phosphatase and bilirubin. WBC is usually normal or slightly low, with a relative lymphocytosis and at times atypical lymphocytes. ESR is normal. Specific serologies are available, and PCR has been helpful in detecting circulating RNA in HCV infection. Liver biopsy may be helpful in clarifying the diagnosis and prognosis in patients who are extremely ill or in those for whom the diagnosis is in doubt.	No specific therapy in acute infection. Interferon may be useful in chronic hepatitis B or hepatitis C infection.

c. Infectious mononucleosis	EB virus is the cause and spreads by the oropharyngeal route. Most overt clinical infections occur in young adults of middle or upper socioeconomic status.	Mild hepatitis is seen in most cases, but marked jaundice is rare. May closely simulate viral hepatitis, but usually marked pharyngitis, adenopathy, and splenomegaly suggest that infectious mononucleosis is more likely.	Marked lymphocytosis and atypical lymphocytes very helpful, though may not appear until second week. Serology very important. If serology negative in this setting, do toxoplasmosis and HIV and CMV titers. Liver function tests frequently show elevation of SGOT and SGPT with milder elevation of bilirubin and alkaline phosphatase.	Symptomatic in vast majority of cases. (corticosteroids may be indicated for laryngeal obstruction and other severe complications such as marked thrombocytopenia, hemolysis, and meningoencephalitis).
d. Leptospirosis	Usually acquired from contact with water or food contaminated by urine from infected animals, especially rats, cattle, swine or dogs.	Jaundice not present in most cases of leptospirosis, but may be marked in some. Common findings include high fever, chills, myalgias, headache, and conjunctival infection. Illness may be diphasic.	Liver function tests are usually abnormal. Bilirubin increases but may be severe and usually elevated more significantly than alkaline phosphatase or SGOT; CPK is frequently elevated. Urine analysis usually abnormal and in many cases shows	Symptomatic. (Antibiotics such as penicillin G and tetracycline are usually given if diagnosis is made early in course of the disease, as they are thought by some to reduce hepatic and renal complications.)

(continued)

TABLE 9.2. *(continued)* DIAGNOSTIC CHART: JAUNDICE-SELECTED ETIOLOGIES

Disease	Etiology, Epidemiology, and/or Pathogenesis	Clinical Signs	Diagnosis	Initial Therapy (Alternative Rx in Parentheses)
			elevated BUN. Serology very helpful. Culture of blood, CSF, and urine on specialized media is rewarding, but growth is slow. CSF shows findings similar to viral meningitis. At times, CSF appears xanthochromic.	
e. Syphilitic hepatitis	Sexually-acquired, usually by homosexual males.	Right-upper quadrant pain, fever, accompanying signs of secondary syphilis, e.g., rash on palms and soles, adenopathy.	RPR, FTA-ABS.	Penicillin (doxycycline).
f. Q fever	Caused by C. burnetii: acquired from inhalation of dust from soil or other materials contaminated by infected livestock. Can also be acquired by drinking contaminated milk.	Jaundice and hepatitis not present in all cases, but may be severe in some. Q fever frequently causes pneumonitis, fever, malaise, and headaches, and conjunctival injection. Unlike other rickettsial infections, rash is very rare.	Serology. Weil-Felix test negative. If liver biopsy done, granulomas frequently present. Most laboratories do not attempt isolation of this highly infectious agent.	Doxycycline (chloramphenicol).

2. Secondary to bloodstream infection: pylephlebitis	Portal venous bacteremia associated with intra-abdominal suppurative process such as appendicitis or diverticulitis.	Hectic fever, chills, right upper quadrant pain and tenderness, and jaundice. Patients usually very sick.	Blood cultures may be positive and WBCs elevated with shift to the left. Liver function tests abnormal. KUB, ultrasound, and CAT scan are usually required to help rule out other right upper quadrant infections and to make this diagnosis. Angiography may be necessary.	Antibiotic combination like Ampicillin-sulbactam plus gentamicin. Surgery.
3. Liver abscess a. Pyogenic	Usually secondary to extrahepatic biliary tract disease, but can be secondary to arterial	Usually marked fever, chills, right upper quadrant pain and tenderness, and jaundice.	Usually WBCs elevated with shift to left. Abnormal liver function tests, especially alkaline	Surgical drainage is usually necessary, but this may be accomplished with a

(continued)

TABLE 9.2. (continued) DIAGNOSTIC CHART: JAUNDICE-SELECTED ETIOLOGIES

Disease	Etiology, Epidemiology, and/or Pathogenesis	Clinical Signs	Diagnosis	Initial Therapy (Alternative Rx in Parentheses)
	bacteremia, portal bacteremia and pylephlebitis, tumor necrosis, penetrating wounds, or abdominal trauma. Abscesses frequently multiple and may occur in any lobe of the liver. May be entirely cryptogenic.	At times, however, the picture may be very subtle and the symptoms mild.	phosphatase. Bilirubin frequently elevated. Blood cultures may be positive. Chest x-ray may show elevated right diaphragm and atelectasis in RLL. KUB may show gas in liver area or gallstone. Ultrasound or CT scan usually diagnostic. At surgery, pus is often foul smelling and Gram stain frequently shows mixture of bacteria. Culture of pus anaerobically and aerobically usually demonstrates bacteria. A search for *E. histolytica* and an amebiasis serology should be pursued to rule out amebiasis.	percutaneous catheter in appropriate patients. Some patients, presumably with early infection, respond to antibiotics alone. Antimicrobial therapy is based on the suspected source of the abscess and cultures taken, results of blood cultures, and results of Gram stain at the time of diagnostic aspiration or surgery. Initial therapy frequently includes regimens like Ampicillin-sulbactam plus an aminoglycoside, to cover the anaerobes, streptococci and Gram-negative enteric bacilli usually associated with this entity.

JAUNDICE

b. Amebic	Secondary to intestinal amebiasis. Evidence of poor sanitation or epidemiologic history of travel to areas of poor sanitation may be helpful.	The illness can resemble a pyogenic abscess, but the patient is usually not as sick and less likely to be jaundiced. Diarrhea may precede liver involvement in a few cases, but is not present in most.	WBCs normal or mildly elevated. Eosinophilia uncommon unless other parasites are present as well. Liver function tests usually show elevation of the alkaline phosphotase and minimal to no elevation of bilirubin. Blood cultures are negative. Chest x-ray usually shows elevated right diaphragm and atelectasis in RLL. Sonogram or CT scan almost always shows evidence of solitary abscess in right lobe. Serology extremely helpful. Stool or rectal biopsy should be examined for ova and parasites. If aspirate of liver abscess is done, the pus found is not foul-smelling and no bacteria are seen. Pus may resemble anchovy paste. Wall of abscess may reveal amebae.	Surgical drainage usually not needed. Antiamebic therapy with metronidazole is followed by a drug effective against intraluminal amebae, e.g., iodoquinol.

10

SPLENOMEGALY

The spleen is the largest aggregate of lymphoid tissue in the body, consisting of a white and a red pulp. The white pulp comprises follicles of plasma cells and lymphocytes with the important function of immunoglobulin synthesis. The red pulp, whose vascular channels are supported by phagocytic cells of the reticuloendothelial system, is responsible for the removal of defective RBCs (culling), RBC inclusions (pitting), microorganisms, and exogenous particulate matter. The spleen frequently enlarges when generalized infection occurs because of increased reticuloendothelial activity and antibody production.

It is difficult to detect splenic enlargement, especially if it is not extreme. The spleen must be enlarged two to four times to be palpable. Therefore, enlargement and palpability are not synonymous. Slight enlargement can sometimes be detected by dullness to percussion of Traube's space, x-rays, or a CT scan. If a left upper quadrant mass is detected, it may represent spleen, but tumors of other organs, e.g., kidney, may present as a left upper quadrant mass resembling splenic enlargement.

It should be noted that a palpable spleen does not always indicate a disease state, since the spleen is normally slightly enlarged in 30 percent of newborns, 15 percent of six-month-olds, and 3 percent of college freshmen. However, once splenic enlargement is detected, the physician must rule out serious disease.

INFECTIOUS CAUSES OF ACUTE SPLENOMEGALY

Infections involving the spleen may be divided into acute, subacute, and chronic illnesses. The most common cause of acute splenomegaly in the United States is infection. In this setting, a nonspecific splenitis, or "acute splenic tumor" occurs. The spleen becomes minimally to moderately enlarged, hyperemic and mushy, and demonstrates reticuloendothelial hyperplasia histologically. Although many microorganisms may cause acute splenomegaly, this finding is more common in certain specific infections. Thus, the presence of splenomegaly helps the clinician in his differential diagnosis (Table 10.1).

Typhoid fever produces a palpable spleen in most patients. The typhoid patient usually exhibits fever, headache, and GI symptoms, and sometimes shows a relative bradycardia, cough, and rose spots. By the end of the first week of illness, the spleen usually becomes palpable, but is soft and may be difficult to appreciate. There may be an audible friction rub over the area of splenic enlargement if infarction is present.

Bacterial endocarditis is more likely to produce splenomegaly when it is subacute (SBE), but acute endocarditis (ABE) also may cause splenic enlargement. Patients with ABE often have a fulminating septic course, with hectic fever and signs of embolization to the periphery or to the lungs. A murmur may not be heard early in the disease. When embolization to the spleen occurs in ABE, a splenic abscess may form, unlike the bland infarcts seen more commonly in SBE. Acute endocarditis often attacks normal heart valves and should be suspected in patients with bacteremia with more virulent organisms, e.g., *S. aureus* and *Streptococcus pneumoniae*. The valves most frequently involved are the aortic and mitral, although tricuspid involvement is also seen and at times is the only site of infection. Drug addicts are especially prone to right-sided ABE because of the contaminated materials they inject into their veins.

A viral illness commonly responsible for acute palpable splenomegaly is infectious mononucleosis. Symptomatic mononucleosis

TABLE 10.1. SPLENOMEGALY

Acute	Subacute/Chronic
1. Bacteremia	1. SBE

Typhoid fever
    ABE
    Other bacteria, somewhat less commonly
	2. Disseminated tuberculosis[a]
	3. Disseminated histoplasmosis[a]

2. Viremia
    Infectious mononucleosis
    Other viruses, including hepatitis, CMV, HHV-6, rubella, HIV (acute)	

3. RMSF, Ehrlichiosis	
4. Psittacosis	
5. Malaria	

Rare Causes of Splenomegaly in the U.S.A.

1. Toxoplasmosis	1. Malaria
2. Secondary syphilis	2. Brucellosis[a]
3. Relapsing fever	3. Congenital syphilis
4. Splenic abscess	4. Chronic meningococcemia
	5. Kala-azar
	6. Schistosomiasis
	7. Echinococcosis[a]
	8. Trypanosomiasis

[a] May produce splenic calcifications.

is seen in young, healthy individuals and presents with fever, sore throat and lymphadenopathy with lymphocytosis. Large numbers of atypical lymphocytes are seen on the peripheral blood smear. The spleen is enlarged in 50 to 75 percent of patients and is largest during the second and third weeks of illness. In this disease, splenic architecture is severely disrupted, and splenic rupture may occur in rare cases. Therefore, frequent and vigorous palpation of the spleen should be avoided. The diagnosis is supported by a positive Monospot (which detects heterophile antibodies), although the most specific serologic test is the detection of Epstein-Barr virus (EBV) antibody.

Occasionally a patient will exhibit a mononucleosis-like illness with a negative Monospot. In these patients the specific EBV serology may establish the diagnosis, although it may occasionally be negative. In this situation, cytomegalovirus (CMV) infection may be the cause of the mononucleosis. CMV typically causes disease in young patients, particularly women, mimicking EBV mononucleosis, but producing less severe pharyngeal inflammation and less prominent cervical adenopathy. CMV also may cause infection in immunocompromised patients, in patients who have had cardiac surgery with bypass, and in recipients of whole blood, leukocyte infusions, and renal, heart, or marrow transplants. Other causes of the mono syndrome include rubella, toxoplasmosis, hepatitis, herpes simplex infection, acute HIV, and the recently-described HHV-6, which is the cause of exanthem subitum (roseola infantum) in infants and may also cause a nonspecific febrile illness in infants and a mono-like illness in the adult.

Rocky Mountain spotted fever is associated with firm, nontender splenomegaly in 50 percent of cases. Patients usually become ill during spring and summer months and present with fever and severe headache. If the patient can provide a reliable history it often includes exposure to a wood or dog tick. The characteristic petechial rash noted on the extremities is not seen for the first few days, and when a rash initially appears, macules suggestive of measles or drug allergy are present rather than the petechiae, which usually appear later in the illness.

In any patient with splenomegaly and acute pneumonia, psittacosis is a consideration. This infection is transmitted to humans by inhalation of dust contaminated with the feces and feathers of infected birds. There may be a severe headache, relative bradycardia, cough, and rarely, red macules (Horder's spots) simulating the rose spots of typhoid fever.

Finally, malaria is an acute illness that frequently causes splenomegaly. Malaria remains a diagnostic consideration in the United States because of increasing international travel and as a result of our economic, cultural, and military involvement in malarious areas of the world. In the United States most patients with malaria have returned from an endemic area where they were infected via the bite of an Anopheles mosquito. Some patients in this country acquire their infection by blood transfusion or by the use of needles shared with a malaria carrier during illicit narcotics injection. The mosquito vector is present in some areas of the United States and is thought to have been responsible for occasional cases. Usually rigors, fever, and anemia are present. Splenic enlargement and tenderness are very common if the illness persists for more than a week. Malaria is the most common cause of spontaneous rupture of the spleen, a complication that occurs most frequently during the initial attack.

CAUSES OF SUBACUTE OR CHRONIC SPLENOMEGALY

Some infectious diseases cause a subacute or chronic splenic enlargement. In these illnesses, the spleen tends to be larger than it is in the acute entities just discussed. Direct infection of the spleen is more likely in this group of patients, and in fact, the etiologic agent is sometimes found within the splenic tissue itself.

SBE is among the more common causes of subacute splenomegaly in the United States. Usually afflicting people with preexisting heart disease, SBE causes a syndrome of weakness, anemia, fever, evolving murmurs, petechiae, and sometimes, deterioration in cardiovascular, neurologic or renal status. The spleen is enlarged in from 25 to 50 percent of cases and is rarely tender except following splenic infarction secondary to embolization from the infected heart valves. In this circumstance, there may be tenderness and an audible rub. Infarcts in SBE are usually bland and

TABLE 10.2. NONINFECTIOUS CAUSES OF SPLENOMEGALY

A. Inflammatory
 1. Felty's syndrome
 2. Sarcoidosis
 3. Berylliosis
 4. Drug hypersensitivity

B. Congestive
 1. Cirrhosis
 2. Portal vein obstruction
 3. Splenic vein obstruction
 4. Congestive heart failure

C. Hyperplastic
 1. Hemolytic anemias
 2. Hemoglobinopathies
 3. Myelophthisic anemia
 4. Systemic lupus erythematous
 5. Thrombotic thrombocytopenic purpura
 6. Grave's disease
 7. Polycythemia vera

D. Infiltrative
 1. Storage diseases (e.g., glycogen)
 2. Amyloidosis
 3. Diabetes mellitus

E. Cysts and neoplasms
 1. Cysts
 2. Hamartomas
 3. Leukemia/lymphoma
 4. Histiocytosis
 5. Metastatic neoplasm

much less likely to progress to abscess formation than are the infarcts seen in ABE. Also, some organisms are more likely to cause abscess than others: for example, splenic abscess is a more frequent complication of enterococcal endocarditis than of other streptococcal endocarditides.

Disseminated tuberculosis is another cause of subacute splenomegaly. This illness may be extremely difficult to diagnose, as patients may show little more than fever and deterioration. The classic miliary pattern found on chest x-ray may not be present, and thus the diagnosis frequently depends on liver or bone marrow biopsy and culture. Although disseminated tuberculosis is usually a fulminant illness, at times it follows a more subacute course; in this latter setting, splenomegaly may be striking. The spleen is actually infected and contains multiple granulomas.

Histoplasmosis produces acute and chronic clinical patterns similar to those produced by tuberculosis. In the chronic disseminated form, splenomegaly is usually present, along with weight loss, anorexia, and fever. Evidence of adrenal insufficiency is present in about one-fifth of these patients. Skin and especially mucous membrane lesions may be present. When such lesions are noted, a biopsy with culture and stains is indicated. Peripheral blood smears and especially bone marrow are important aids to diagnosis. *H. capsulatum* may be seen in the macrophages at these two sites, and the organisms are frequently grown from bone marrow. It should be remembered that half of the cases of disseminated histoplasmosis show no pulmonary involvement, although the lung is the most likely primary site of infection.

Several causes of chronic splenic enlargement are important in other countries. A geographical history is particularly important in leading the clinician to the consideration of diseases such as kala-azar, schistosomiasis, echinococcosis, trypanosomiasis, and of course, chronic malaria.

Of the many infectious causes of splenic calcification, histoplasmosis is the most frequent. Echinococcosis, tuberculosis, and brucellosis are also considerations.

Although this discussion is concerned with specific infections that cause splenomegaly, it is important to keep in mind that many noninfectious diseases that cause splenomegaly (Table 10.2) are frequently complicated by fever with or without infection. For example, a patient with lymphoma may present with the syndrome of splenomegaly and fever; in this case, the fever may be induced by the neoplastic process or may indicate an associated infection. Splenomegaly may also accompany fever and a "mononucleosis-like" illness as a result of drug hypersensitivity, e.g., to Dilantin.

TABLE 10.3. DIAGNOSTIC CHART: SPLENOMEGALY—SELECTED ETIOLOGIES

Disease	Epidemiology and/or Pathogenesis	Clinical Signs	Diagnosis	Initial Treatment
A. Miliary tuberculosis	Usually spread from reactivation of pulmonary lesions with massive spread to bloodstream. May also result from overwhelming primary infection, especially in the young.	May have severe hypoxia, fever, hematologic abnormalities, abnormal liver function. Chest x-rays may not show the miliary pattern early. Choroid tubercles are common, and evidence of meningeal tuberculosis may be present. Spleen is enlarged in 10–15%. Splenic calcification may result from tuberculosis.	Chest x-ray. Sputum smear and culture (may be positive or negative). Marrow and liver biopsy and culture. Skin test may be positive or negative. CSF may show evidence of granulomatous meningitis.	Isoniazid + rifampin + ethambutol + pyrazinamide. Corticosteroids may be indicated for severe hypoxia or for tuberculous meningitis.
B. Disseminated histoplasmosis	Results from activation of prior pulmonary focus or from progression of initial lesion.	Fever, subacute to acute deterioration. Lesions of tongue and mucous membranes may be present and are helpful clinical clues and	Culture of blood and especially bone marrow. Smear and stains of sputum, blood, bone marrow, skin, and mucous membrane lesions. Look	Amphotericin B.

SPLENOMEGALY

		rewarding biopsy sites. Splenomegaly and generalized adenopathy commonly seen. Splenic calcifications common, but occur late.	for organisms in phagocytes. Skin test not helpful clinically and may make serology difficult to interpret. Serology.	
C. Malaria	In U.S., usually imported from malarious areas in other parts of the world. Infection in the US may be transmitted by blood transfusion or by contaminated needles shared among drug abusers. Very rarely cases occur in the U.S. that are related to infected mosquitoes. Large areas of the US do have the appropriate Anopheles mosquito vector present.	Fever (at times relapsing) and chills. Hemolytic anemia may be present. Tender splenomegaly very common. WBC usually normal. Faciparum malaria may produce severe cerebritis, pneumonia, and massive hemolysis.	Thin and thick smears of peripheral blood during febrile episodes. Most clinicians not used to dealing with malaria are more likely to make diagnosis from thin smears, although experienced microbiologists prefer thick smears. Stain with Wright's or Giemsa. Smears should be verified by state health lab or C.D.C.	Chloroquine: if chloroquine resistant *P. falciparum* suspected use quinine and doxycycline or quinine and Clindamycin. If patient is severely ill, use IV quinidine and clindamycin.

(continued)

TABLE 10.3. (continued)

Disease	Epidemiology and/or Pathogenesis	Clinical Signs	Diagnosis	Initial Treatment
D. Infectious mononucleosis	EBV is present in the oropharynx for a long duration after clinical episode. Spread thought to result from pharyngeal carriers. This clinical entity can be mimicked by other viruses such as CMV, herpes simplex, HIV, adenovirus and hepatitis viruses as well as by toxoplasma.	Most disease is asymptomatic or very mild. Symptomatic infection in adolescents and young adults consists of fever, sore throat, adenopathy, supraorbital edema, and splenomegaly. Hepatitis is common. A maculopapular rash is rare, but if ampicillin is given, 90% of patients will show a rash. Various neurologic syndromes are also seen. The spleen is enlarged in 50–70% of cases, especially during the second and third weeks. Death from splenic rupture is rare, but occurs.	Increased numbers of lymphocytes with many atypical lymphs common on peripheral blood smear. Serology helpful: Monospot, which detects heterophile antibodies, and the more specific anti-EBV antibodies.	Treatment is rarely needed, but corticosteroids may be used for the complications of laryngeal edema hemolysis, thrombocytopenia, and meningoencephalitis.

E. Typhoid fever	Causative organism is *S. typhi*. Spread is by food or water that has been contaminated by excreta of a human carrier. The asymptomatic chronic carrier is an important host in the U.S. Flies can be vectors, and water can contaminate shellfish. Occasionally other salmonellae may produce an enteric fever that can mimic *S. typhi* infection.	Headache, fever, constipation, bradycardia, rose spots, and leukopenia are common. A soft, enlarged spleen is often seen. At times diarrhea noted instead of constipation.	Culture blood, urine, stool rose spots. If negative, culture bone marrow. Stool smear may show many mononuclear cells; serology helpful.	Depending on sensitivities, may be TMP/SMX, ciprofloxacin or ceftriaxone. Some still prefer chloramphenicol.

(continued)

TABLE 10.3. (continued)

Disease	Epidemiology and/or Pathogenesis	Clinical Signs	Diagnosis	Initial Treatment
F. Infective endocarditis	Acute: Patient may or may not have history of significant valvular heart disease. Frequently occurs during bacteremia with S. aureus, but at times with enterococci or with Gram-negative rods. Lesions are usually aortic or mitral, but tricuspid involvement is common in intravenous drug abusers. Subacute: Patients with rheumatic, arteriosclerotic, congenital heart disease and mitral valve prolapse at risk, often after bacteremia with organisms of low virulence. Prosthetic: Patients with prosthetic heart valves are also at very high risk, both at time of surgery and during episodes of bacteremia	Fever, murmur, microscopic hematuria, petechiae, and heart failure. Splenomegaly in subacute cases. Spleen rarely tender unless infarct is present; then may have rub and tenderness. Rarely splenic abscess may form, especially with acute disease. Acute endocarditis is much less likely to cause splenomegaly and may even present without a murmur. In recent years endocarditis has tended to present without classic features.	Blood cultures are positive in 85% if 5 separate specimens are drawn; more than 5 sets of cultures give few additional positives. Positive rheumatoid factor in 50% of patients who have had disease longer than 6 weeks. Low serum complement if nephritis present. Elevated ESR common lab abnormality. Gram stain and culture emboli if embolectomy done (especially good for fungal endocarditis). If blood cultures are negative, perform fungal serology, Q fever serology; inoculate small amounts of blood to dilute serum antibody, do buffy coat smear, culture for nutritionally-deficient	Unknown organism, acute endocarditis: Vancomycin or Nafcillin plus gentamicin. Unknown organism, subacute endocarditis: ampicillin plus gentamicin. Unknown organism; prosthetic valve endocarditis: vancomycin and gentamicin ± rifampin.

SPLENOMEGALY

	after surgery.	and cell-wall deficient organisms, and discuss with the microbiologist any additional media or cultural techniques that could be attempted. Echocardiogram more helpful in identifying complications than in making the diagnosis.		
G. Psittacosis	Aerosol spread of dust contaminated with feces of infected birds, especially parakeets, parrots, and turkeys.	Intense headache, fever, cough, and Horder's spots. Splenomegaly seen in 10–70%. Chest x-ray may show patchy areas of infiltration or lobar consolidation.	Serology helpful.	Doxycycline. (erythromycin)
H. Rocky Mountain spotted fever	Organism is *Rickettsia rickettsiae*; spread by dog or wood tick. Most frequent in the Southeast US but seen in most regions, predominantly in summer and fall.	Fever, severe headache, and macular rash, which usually becomes petechial. Rash begins peripherally, sometimes involving the palms and soles. Splenomegaly present in 50%; spleen is firm, nontender.	Serology helpful. Decreased platelets common. May show DIC. WBC is low, normal, or high, but usually shows an increase in bands. LP can show mild pleocytosis. Biopsy of skin lesions may show rickettsiae in areas of vasculitis with special stains, e.g., direct immunofluorescence or immunoperoxidase.	Doxycycline. (chloramphenicol)

11

LOCALIZED AND GENERALIZED LYMPHADENOPATHY

The filtration of microorganisms, the production of antibody, and the processing of lymphocytes are a few of the important roles played by the 600 lymph nodes in the human body. With the exception of neoplasia, lymph nodes are rarely the site of primary disease. However, they are involved in virtually all infectious processes. When a local infection occurs, regional lymph node reaction is usually demonstrable. If this barrier of host resistance is overcome, the infectious process may spread to more distant nodes or to the blood stream. At times, generalized lymphadenopathy and reticuloendothelial system (RES) hyperplasia occur secondary to widespread sepsis.

Lymphadenopathy can be categorized as (a) acute or chronic, (b) local or generalized, and (c) with or without specific histology. Most patients who present with lymphadenopathies have acute, localized processes, and biopsy of the involved nodes shows nonspecific histology, i.e., regional nonspecific lymphadenitis.

Acutely inflamed nodes become enlarged because of cellular infiltration and edema, and if capsular distension is marked, tenderness is present. The nodes may become fluctuant if invaded by bacteria. Fluctuance may also occur in nonbacterial infections such as lymphogranuloma venereum (LGV).

TABLE 11.1. LOCALIZED AND GENERALIZED LYMPHADENOPATHY

A. Localized lymphadenopathy
  1. Cervical adenopathy
     a. Pharyngitis
        (1) Viral (mono, others)
        (2) Bacterial (group A strep, fusospirochetal, diphtheria, Yersinia, gonococcus, A. hemolyticum)
        (3) Mycoplasma
     b. Mycobacterial adenitis
     c. MLNS (Kawasaki disease)
  2. Occipital adenopathy
     a. Nonspecific scalp infection
     b. Rubella
  3. Peripheral adenopathy
     a. Location varies with inoculation site
        (1) Bacterial adenitis (caused by streptococcus and other pyogens)
        (2) Cat-scratch disease
        (3) Tularemia
        (4) Plague
        (5) Rat-bite fever (S. minus)
     b. Usually axillary or epitrochlear
        (1) Sporotrichosis
        (2) Herpes zoster infection
        (3) Herpetic whitlow
     c. Usually inguinal (ulcer-adenopathy syndrome)
        (1) Primary syphilis
        (2) LGV
        (3) Chancroid
        (4) Granuloma inguinale
        (5) Genital herpes infection (herpes hominis, type II)

B. Generalized lymphadenopathy
  1. Mono syndrome (EBV, rubella, CMV, toxo, HIV, hepatitis, HHV-6)
  2. Measles
  3. Dengue
  4. Tularemia
  5. Brucellosis
  6. Tuberculosis
  7. Histoplasmosis
  8. Secondary syphilis
  9. HIV infection

Chronic inflammation is frequently manifested by enlarged nodes, with mononuclear cell infiltration and relative preservation of normal architecture. The changes seen on lymph node biopsy may be nonspecific, preventing an exact diagnosis. Even the presence of epithelioid granulomas with caseous necrosis and giant-cell formation is not in itself diagnostic of tuberculosis, since the same findings may be seen in tularemia, LGV, cat-scratch disease, brucellosis, and even sarcoidosis. With appropriate cultures and stains such as Ziehl-Neelsen, PAS, and the Gomori silver stain, a specific microorganism may occasionally be identified.

In the following discussion, adenopathy is categorized as localized, according to specific anatomic regions, or as generalized (Table 11.1).

LOCAL ADENOPATHY

Although the classification of localized lymphadenopathy at different body sites is clinically useful, it is important to recognize that exceptions occur. For example, the sexually transmitted disorders usually affect the genitalia and inguinal lymph nodes, but if the primary lesion (e.g., a syphilitic chancre) is located elsewhere, e.g., the mouth, the adenopathy will be in the cervical area. Similarly, diseases spread by insect vectors will cause adenopathy in the area corresponding to the site of inoculation. Therefore, depending on the location of the bite, local anatomy will determine which nodes are involved.

Cervical Adenitis

Cervical adenitis is usually secondary to pharyngitis of viral or streptococcal etiology. Group A streptococcal infection (*Streptococcus pyogenes*) of the pharynx can cause tender anterior cervical adenopathy. The appearance of the pharynx, the presence of exudative material, and the character of the nodes are all nonspecific. The clinician is not able to identify the specific etiology on purely clinical grounds.

Infectious mononucleosis is usually associated with a pharyngitis that may be exudative. Cervical adenitis involving both the anterior and posterior cervical nodes is almost always present.

Mononucleosis especially should be considered as a cause of pharyngitis in the adolescent or young adult. The lymphadenopathy may not be localized to just the cervical region but may be generalized, and splenomegaly, palatal petechiae, supraorbital edema, and a generalized maculopapular rash may occur. If ampicillin is given because of suspected bacterial infection, 90 percent of patients with EBV (Epstein-Barr virus) infectious mononucleosis will develop a generalized nonpruritic maculopapular eruption, which is not thought to represent ampicillin allergy. Evidence of hepatomegaly and/or abnormalities of liver function are very common in infectious mononucleosis. Diagnosis is usually made readily by evaluation of the peripheral blood smear and by serologic studies.

On occasion, disease due to cytomegalovirus (CMV) infection or to acquired toxoplasmosis can mimic infectious mononucleosis, but the Monospot and EBV antibody determinations are negative. The pharyngitis and cervical adenopathy in CMV infection is less pronounced than in EBV mononucleosis.

The pharyngitis seen with infectious mononucleosis and streptococcal disease is difficult to distinguish clinically from many other viral pharyngitides. Adenovirus and herpes simplex type 1 can produce particularly severe exudative and ulcerative pharyngitis, as can primary HIV infection. Mycoplasma may cause a mild pharyngitis similar to viral infection. Occasional bacterial etiologies of pharyngitis include gonococcal infection (severe pain but minimal erythema, and failure to respond to usual treatment for pharyngitis), *A. hemolyticum* (may be accompanied by a diffuse erythema) and Yersinia (sometimes suggested by gastrointestinal symptomatology).

In cervical adenitis due to atypical mycobacteria, the node enlargement is usually unilateral and isolated to one group of nodes, with no evidence of disease elsewhere. This syndrome is typically seen in children from 2 to 8 years of age who are otherwise healthy and have a negative chest x-ray. The responsible pathogens are most likely *M. scrofulaceum* and *M. avium complex* (MAC). Mycobacterial cervical adenitis in young adults, aged 20 to 40, is usually caused by classical *M. tuberculosis*. In these cases, active tuberculosis is usually present elsewhere in the body, although the chest x-ray may show no evidence of tuberculosis in 50 per cent of patients.

Lymph nodes in mycobacterial infections may be large and matted together and are usually painless. The course of tuberculous adenitis is generally chronic. Although the finding of caseating granulomata is helpful, it is not diagnostic unless the organisms can be found. Specimens for cultures must be taken at the time of excision or biopsy not only to identify the presence of mycobacteria, but also to classify them. The tuberculin skin test is helpful but in no way replaces biopsy with culture. Tuberculous adenopathy caused by *M. tuberculosis* usually responds to antituberculous therapy alone, but excision is generally required to treat disease caused by atypical mycobacteria.

An extremely rare cause of acute cervical lymphadenopathy is diphtheria. In some areas of the country, low levels of immunity exist, so that a history of immunization is crucial in the evaluation of a patient with symptoms consistent with diphtheria. Difficult to recognize except in an epidemic situation, diphtheria should be suspected in any nonimmunized patient with a pharyngitis accompanied by a gray pseudomembrane that is difficult to remove. Cervical adenopathy and edema of the anterior neck and submandibular areas frequently occur with this form of pharyngitis. In the hands of an experienced bacteriologist, a methylene blue smear of the membrane reveals myriads of Gram-positive rods with characteristic morphology, but this technique should never be relied on for the diagnosis. Diphtheria should be diagnosed purely on the basis of the clinical and epidemiologic history and on physical findings. Antitoxin should be given immediately if the clinical presentation is highly suggestive of this diagnosis, if the patient has not previously been completely immunized. Cultures should be positive in Loeffler's medium within 12 hours, unless the patient has received antibiotics. Other much more frequent causes of a pharyngeal pseudomembrane are infectious mononucleosis, streptococcosis, fusospirochetal infection, candidiasis, and a variety of upper respiratory viral pathogens.

The mucocutaneous lymph node syndrome (MLNS or Kawasaki disease) is characterized by protracted fever (longer than five days) associated with cervical adenopathy, conjunctival injection, redness of pharynx and lips, and diffuse scarlatiniform rash including the palms and soles, with later desquamation. The disease may be mistaken for Group A streptococcal scarlet fever, but the diagnostic studies for streptococcal infection are negative and penicillin is not helpful. The etiology of MLNS is unknown; the fatality rate (about 1 percent) is related to coronary arteritis. High dose aspirin and gamma globulin are helpful therapeutically.

Cervical adenopathy may be simulated by other inflammatory processes of the neck, for example, parotitis and Ludwig's angina.

Occipital Lymphadenopathy

Occipital lymphadenopathy has many causes. Local infections of the scalp such as pediculosis capitis, impetigo, and ringworm may be responsible. Systemic infections like syphilis and tuberculosis may enlarge occipital nodes, but usually involve other nodes more dramatically and are discussed elsewhere. A common generalized infection that especially involves occipital nodes is rubella, and this adenopathy may precede the rubella rash by several days. In rubella the nodes, although generalized, usually predominate in occipital, mastoid, and posterior cervical locations. They are never huge and only rarely tender. This pattern of adenopathy, together with rash, fever, and upper respiratory symptoms, may also be seen in rubeola.

Peripheral Axillary, Epitrochlear, and Inguinal Adenopathy

Many infections predictably affect either the epitrochlear and axillary or the inguinal lymph nodes, because their primary lesion is nearly always located on the upper or lower extremity, respectively. However, there is a group of infections whose epidemiology is variable enough that the site of inoculation is not predictable, so that enlargement of either axillary or inguinal nodes may result. This latter group will be discussed first.

Enlargement of the axillary and epitrochlear or inguinal nodes occurs most frequently from infection on the extremities with pyogenic organisms. Such infections may be acute or quite indolent. The repeated trauma to the lower extremities that we all encounter is sufficient to enlarge the inguinal nodes. Since a minor degree of nonspecific inguinal adenopathy is present in so many people, biopsy of the inguinal nodes is a relatively unrewarding diagnostic maneuver. If other nodes are enlarged and accessible, they are preferred for biopsy.

Group A streptococcal infection of the extremities may produce cellulitis and lymphangitis with regional adenopathy, with or without an obvious source. Any extremity may be involved. Fever and superficial red streaks may occur, with painful and tender swollen regional nodes. At times the adenitis may be "primary," without evidence of a peripheral site of infection. Bacteria other than streptococci are occasionally etiologic.

Tularemia of the ulceroglandular type is most frequently associated with the bite of a tick or deerfly, or with contact with the carcass of an infected animal. The site of inoculation is characterized by an ulcerating papule. Regional adenopathy, the location of which depends on the inoculation site, is manifested by hot, large, fluctuant, and tender lymph nodes that may suppurate and drain spontaneously. On the other hand, the node enlargement may at times be much less dramatic and recognized only after very careful physical examination.

Among the less common but important causes of localized adenitis in the epitrochlear, axillary, and inguinal areas is cat-scratch disease, which results one to three weeks after being licked or scratched on the extremity by an infected cat. Facial lesions may be associated with cervical or auricular adenopathy. At times, however, no history of cat contact is obtained. The primary lesion that is observed in the majority of cases is a tender papule that is frequently capped by a vesicle. Regional nodes then become enlarged and tender, and the overlying skin may be red. Constitutional signs are usually mild. If the node becomes fluctuant, it should be aspirated but not incised. This procedure will reduce local pain and may effect a dramatic lysis of fever.

A cat-scratch skin test has been helpful in the past, and now the etiology of cat-scratch disease has been shown to be bacterial, due to *Bartonella* (formerly *Rochalimaea*) *henselae*. Silver stains of a node biopsy show characteristic organisms. If available, cultural techniques can grow the etiologic agent and PCR can sometimes detect its presence.

Plague is a rare human disease in the United States, but is endemic in rodents in the Southwest. It is usually spread to humans by the bite of a rat flea on the arm or leg. The individuals at particular risk are those living in the endemic area and those whose lifestyle places them in close contact with infected fleas.

The most common form of disease, bubonic plague, is manifested by high fever and severe systemic toxicity, as well as by an erythematous, edematous matted group of inguinal or axillary nodes that can suppurate and drain spontaneously. The inoculating flea bite is usually not apparent. The bubo, which is extremely tender, may be aspirated for diagnosis. Sometimes fever regresses temporarily when the bubo first appears.

Rat-bite fever caused by *S. minus* may also cause the syndrome of localized adenopathy, a peripheral lesion on the extremity, and fever. The illness is most frequently seen in infants and young children. One to four weeks after the bite, the local lesion flares once again as the major systemic phase of the illness begins. Fever, generalized rash, and arthritis occur. The local infected nodes are tender, firm, and freely movable. In the other form of rat-bite fever, caused by *S. moniliformis*, adenopathy is not prominent.

Other infections that primarily enlarge epitrochlear and axillary nodes are sporotrichosis, herpes zoster, and herpetic whitlow.

Sporotrichum schenkii usually afflicts people who work with plants, causing a primary lesion of the hand and the characteristic intermittent hard red lumps along the lymphatics. The regional nodes then enlarge and the cutaneous nodules may ulcerate. Pain and fever are absent, and the streaking seen in acute bacterial lymphangitis is rare. Sporotrichosis is definitively diagnosed by culture of the nodules, since neither serology nor scrapings of the lesions for staining are especially helpful. Usually the infection stays localized but requires a long time for resolution. Treatment with a saturated solution of potassium iodide accelerates the clinical response. Although rare, primary cutaneous coccidioidomycosis, nocardiosis, and blastomycosis may mimic this type of local sporotrichosis. These diseases may be diagnosed by biopsy with appropriate stains and cultures.

Most commonly seen on the trunk, herpes zoster causes a syndrome of clustered vesicles in a unilateral segmental distribution, frequently preceded and accompanied by marked paresthesias, mild fever, and headache. These latter signs and symptoms usually precede the rash by a few days but at times by as long as one to two weeks. Regional adenitis is a consistent feature of herpes zoster. The nodes are nontender and freely movable.

Epitrochlear and axillary adenopathy may be a complication of herpetic whitlow, an infection of the pulp of a finger caused by herpes simplex, usually type I. At high risk for this infection are nurses, dentists, and their assistants, who are exposed to herpetic infections in the mouths of patients. This primary lesion is usually very painful.

Inguinal Adenopathy Caused by Sexually Transmitted Diseases

Many sexually transmitted infections are responsible for inguinal lymph node enlargement. Frequently, a genital ulcer accompanies the adenopathy, producing the "ulcer-adenopathy" syndrome. A painless chancre, usually on the external genitalia, with enlarged, freely movable, firm, nonsuppurating, and painless inguinal lymph nodes is characteristic of primary syphilis. Although the initial lesion heals in two to six weeks, the nodes may persist for months. Diagnosis of primary syphilis is made by a characteristic lesion and serology.

Unlike syphilis, the genital ulcers and inguinal nodes of chancroid are tender and painful. If untreated, the nodes may suppurate and rupture to form a large single ulcer. This last complication may be prevented by aspiration when the node is tense. The aspirate may then be smeared and cultured for diagnosis. Biopsy and stains from the undermined edge of the ulcer may also be of assistance.

Inguinal adenopathy is very prominent in LGV and may progress to multilocular suppuration with multiple fistulae. At times the inguinal ligament forms a line of cleavage through the matted nodes, which are enlarged both above and below the ligament (the "Groove" sign). Though this relationship is said to be characteristic of LGV, it is observed only occasionally and is not pathognomonic. The primary genital lesion is a single small ulceration that generally goes unnoticed. It has usually disappeared by the time the lymph node enlargement occurs. Rarely, the primary lesions may occur on the face or finger, and then the node involvement will be appropriately regional. LGV may be accompanied by generalized constitutional symptoms and is occasionally associated with severe arthralgias, diarrhea, and hyperglobulinemia.

The diagnosis is usually made from clinical appearance and appropriate serological studies.

Granuloma inguinale is rare in the United States. The disease is manifested by a painless genital papule or nodule that erodes to leave a beefy red granular base. The infection spreads to the inguinal area and produces a marked subcutaneous swelling. The lesion is called a "pseudobubo," since it is not really due to lymph node involvement, but rather to soft tissue granulation and frequently ulceration. Biopsy or impression smears from the edge of the lesions is diagnostic if cells filled with "Donovan bodies" are seen.

Genital herpetic lesions are characteristically multiple, small erosions on an erythematous base, typically arranged in a cluster. They are extremely painful and are often accompanied by bilateral or unilateral inguinal adenopathy.

GENERALIZED ADENOPATHY

Fever and generalized adenopathy, when caused by infection, are usually due to viral disease, especially EBV mononucleosis and rubella. Other causes include disseminated tuberculosis, secondary syphilis, toxoplasmosis, tularemia, and brucellosis. A good epidemiologic history is helpful in suggesting the specific etiologic diagnosis.

Of the viruses that cause generalized lymphadenopathy, EBV mononucleosis and rubella are very frequent and were discussed earlier as important causes of regional adenitis. EBV mononucleosis may also be simulated by infection with CMV, toxoplasma and HIV. Acquired or reactivated CMV infection is most frequent in normal young people, in patients who have had surgery with bypass (postperfusion syndrome), recipients of blood transfusions, leukocyte infusions and transplants, and in immunocompromised individuals. Patients with this syndrome may present with protracted fever and with moderate hepatic inflammation along with lymphocytosis and atypical lymphocytes, which occur late in the course of the disease. Splenomegaly and adenopathy are not always present. The serologic response is late. The virus may be isolated in the urine and the blood. Other viruses, particularly rubella, adenovirus, and dengue cause significant generalized lymph node enlargement on occasion. Primary HIV infection causes a mono-like illness often accompanied by a diffuse salmon-colored rash that includes the palms and soles. Later in the course of HIV infection generalized adenopathy may return as the infection becomes more advanced.

A history of eating improperly cooked meat or of exposure to cats may be a clue to the diagnosis of toxoplasmosis in a patient with unexplained generalized lymphadenopathy and fever. The most common syndrome seen in acquired symptomatic toxoplasmosis resembles EBV mononucleosis, with enlarged nonsuppurative lymph nodes, fever, and maculopapular rash. The nodes in toxoplasmosis are firm, discreet, freely movable, and at times, painful and tender. Histologic examination of these nodes is considered by some pathologists to be highly characteristic for toxoplasmosis. The disease has on occasion been misdiagnosed as Hodgkin's disease. Frequently the cervical nodes are the largest, increasing the clinical similarity of this entity to mononucleosis. Toxoplasmosis may at times significantly involve the CNS, liver, heart, lungs, or eyes as target organs. This infection must be especially considered in patients with an underlying disease such as lymphoma. When toxoplasmosis occurs in pregnancy, consultation with an infectious diseases specialist is advisable to discuss indications for abortion or medical therapy to prevent the potential serious fetal complications.

Other mimics of the mono syndrome include Hepatitis and infection with HHV-6, which is the etiology of roseola infantum and may cause a mono-like illness in the adult.

Brucellosis should be suspected in individuals who have direct contact with farm animals or dogs (especially beagles), or who ingest unpasteurized milk or milk products. Most of the patients today are abattoir workers. Fever, chills, hepatosplenomegaly, depression, arthralgia, and leukopenia with relative lymphocytosis are commonly noted and are accompanied by small, non-tender, cervical and axillary node enlargement. These nodes may show granulomas or a striking reticuloendothelial hyperplasia with some multinucleate giant cells. Testicular swelling and/or pain may occur. The diagnosis can usually be made by blood or bone marrow cultures and seroconversion.

Disseminated histoplasmosis and other deep fungal infections are capable of producing widespread lymphadenopathy as part of the generalized reticuloendothelial reaction to these agents.

Secondary syphilis is recognized by nontender, generalized lymphadenopathy with fever and a diffuse nonpruritic maculopapular rash, which often includes the palms and soles. The nodes may remain palpable even months after the disappearance of other stigmata of secondary syphilis, i.e., fever, rash, condylomata, and mucous patches. Pre and postauricular, occipital and epitrochlear nodes are all frequently enlarged in secondary syphilis. Serology (VDRL or FTA) is almost invariably positive at this stage of the disease.

Miliary TB may cause generalized adenopathy. At times the typical miliary pattern on chest x-ray may be delayed.

A final note of caution is in order. The combination of fever and adenopathy does not always indicate a single disease process. For example, many noninfectious disorders include adenopathy among their manifestations, e.g., lymphoreticular malignancies, SLE (systemic lupus erythematosus), etc. (Table 11.2). These disorders may cause fever, producing a syndrome of fever and adenopathy that is not infectious in etiology. In addition, some of these noninfectious lymphopathic diseases may be complicated by infection.

TABLE 11.2. NONINFECTIOUS CAUSES OF LOCALIZED AND GENERALIZED LYMPHADENOPATHY

A. Neoplasms
   1. Lymphoreticular malignancies
   2. Paraproteinemias
   3. Metastatic disease

B. Collagen-vascular disorders
   1. Rheumatoid arthritis
   2. Juvenile rheumatoid arthritis
   3. Systemic lupus erythematous

C. Hypersensitivity states
   1. Serum sickness
   2. Drugs, e.g., Dilantin, INH, etc.

D. Miscellaneous
   1. Sarcoidosis
   2. Hyperthyroidism
   3. Autoimmune hemolytic anemia
   4. Histocytosis X
   5. Exfoliative dermatitis
   6. Amyloidosis
   7. Kikuchi Fujimoto disease

TABLE 11.3. DIAGNOSTIC CHART: LOCALIZED AND GENERALIZED LYMPHADENOPATHY—SELECTED ETIOLOGIES

Disease	Epidemiology, Etiology, and/or Pathogenesis	Clinical Signs	Diagnosis	Initial Treatment (Alternate Rx in Parentheses)
A. Localized lymphadenopathy				
1. Cervical adenopathy				
a. Pharyngitis				
1) Viral (nonspecific)	Many different viruses such as adenovirus, enterovirus, parainfluenza, primary HIV, herpes simplex, and others cause pharyngitis and adenitis.	Short-lived illness with sore throat, fever, and tender adenopathy; difficult to differentiate from streptococcal pharyngitis clinically. Vesicular lesions in the pharynx may be present with some of these viral infections.	Usually by excluding streptococcal pharyngitis by culture. May do viral culture and serologies in selected instances.	Supportive.
2) Group A streptococcal	Caused by group A B-hemolytic streptococci.	Symptoms as above. At times marked difficulty swallowing. Exudative	Throat culture; serology used only rarely to help document prior	Penicillin G (erythromycin). Ten days of adequate

LOCALIZED AND GENERALIZED LYMPHADENOPATHY

3) Infectious mononucleosis	EBV spreads infection via oropharyngeal route. Virus may be present in pharynx months after infection occurs.	pharyngitis frequently seen with streptococcal infection but may be caused by many viruses, including EBV. Most clinically significant cases occur in adolescents and young adults, causing fever, sore throat, and anterior and posterior cervical lymphadenopathy. May also see palatal petechiae, splenomegaly, supraorbital edema, and maculopapular rash. A pseudo-membrane may be noted in the pharynx causing confusion with diphtheria.	streptococcal pharyngitis. Several rapid tests available to detect streptococcal antigen on swabs. Lymphocytosis with many atypical cells seen in peripheral smear; also may be noted on a pharyngeal swab. Significant anemia rare. Serology very helpful. Abnormal LFTs frequent. If serology negative for infectious mononucleosis, do serology for hepatitis, HIV, toxoplasmosis, CMV, and other suspected viruses. At times group A streptococci may be isolated from the throat of patients with infectious mononucleosis.	chemotherapy required. Supportive in most cases. Corticosteroids are helpful for laryngeal obstruction.

(continued)

TABLE 11.3. *(continued)*

Disease	Epidemiology, Etiology, and/or Pathogenesis	Clinical Signs	Diagnosis	Initial Treatment (Alternate Rx in Parentheses)
4) Diphtheria	Droplet transmission from pharyngeal carriers or occasionally from an active case. Skin lesions may also service as important reservoirs of infection and have been responsible for recent outbreaks in vagrants. Fomites and dust may be important vehicles for transmission.	Severe cases seen only in unimmunized individuals. Pharyngeal grey pseudomembrane (mimicked by infectious mononucleosis, streptococci, some viruses, fusospirochetal infection, Candida). Minimal pharyngeal discomfort. May see enlargement of cervical nodes, edema of anterior neck, and submandibular areas (bull neck). Severe laryngeal involvement may occur. Complications: myocarditis, peripheral or cranial nerve palsies. A helpful clue is asymmetry	Culture on special media, e.g., Loeffler's. Methylene blue smear helpful in experienced hands.	Antitoxin (give as soon as diagnosis is suspected). Erythromycin to prevent spread and further toxin production.

		of the pharyngeal exudate, especially if it includes soft palate and uvula.		
5) Yersinia	Not clear. Probably secondary to G-I infection.	Exudative pharyngitis, sometimes without G-I symptoms	Culture.	Bactrim, Ciprofloxacin.
6) Gonococcus	Oro-genital sexual contact.	Severe pain, often with only slight erythema. Failure to respond to usual Rx for pharyngitis.	Culture.	Ceftriaxone Ciprofloxacin
7) A. hemolyticum	Probably respiratory spread	Exudative pharyngitis with generalized erythema.	Culture	?erythromycin.
8) Fusospirochetal infection	Necrotizing infection of gingiva, buccal mucosa, or pharynx (especially tonsils) caused by mixture of fusobacteria and spirochetes, hence the term fusospirochetal. Associated with malnutrition, poor oral hygiene. Sometimes the pharyngitis is called Vincent's angina.	Erythematous ulcerations sometimes covered by grey pseudomembrane. Breath has offensive odor.	Gram stain of ulcerations shows mixed flora and PMLs.	Mouth rinse, e.g., with H_2O_2; improved oral hygiene; Clindamycin (Amoxicillin-clavulanate).

(continued)

TABLE 11.3. *(continued)*

Disease	Epidemiology, Etiology, and/or Pathogenesis	Clinical Signs	Diagnosis	Initial Treatment (Alternate Rx in Parentheses)
b. Mycobacterial adenitis	*M. tuberculosis:* usually part of a generalized infection. Atypical mycobacteria: epidemiology unclear; seen mostly in children.	Nodes may be painless or painful, and may become fluctuant, causing draining sinuses. *M. tuberculosis:* multiple groups of nodes involved, frequently bilateral. May see evidence of TB elsewhere. Atypical mycobacteria: usually in children; nodes are unilateral, usually 1 group enlarged. Usually see no evidence of disease elsewhere. Negative contact history.	Chest x-ray. Skin test. Smear and culture of sputum, culture of gastrics, and skin tests; note biopsy shows wide spectrum: giant cells, tubercles, caseous necrosis, fibrosis, calcification; lesions identical to those seen in other organs. Node must be cultured, as organisms are difficult to visualize.	*M. tuberculosis:* Isoniazid + rifampin + ethambutol + pyrazinamide; surgery needed only for diagnosis and for drainage of cold abscess. Atypical mycobacteria: excision is usually curative. If antibacterial agents are used, sensitivities should be known, since resistance is common.

LOCALIZED AND GENERALIZED LYMPHADENOPATHY

c. MLNS (Kawasaki disease)	Usually in children. Specific etiology not known.	Fever not responsive to antibiotics, conjunctival injection, "strawberry" tongue, erythematous rash, cervical adenopathy, desquamation from fingertips. Usually self-limited, but mortality (from coronary arteritis) seen in 1–2%.	Clinical presentation; failure to prove another specific etiology, particularly streptococcal.	Aspirin, immune serum globulin.
2. Occipital adenopathy				
a. Nonspecific scalp infection	Local trauma or infected insect bites. Organisms usually staphylococci or streptococci	Local signs of inflammation.	Clinical presentation. Culture and Gram stain of infected site.	Antibiotics as per Gram stain, culture, and sensitivity.
b. Rubella	Nasopharyngeal secretions are infectious. If disease occurs in pregnancy, products of conception are infectious and congenital rubella infection requires strict isolation.	Fever, faint pink macular rash; adenopathy; back of neck, especially along sternomastoid, around the mastoid, and in suboccipital locations. Adenopathy may be generalized. Nodes are small and only rarely tender; they may precede the rash.	Serology helpful. Virus may be isolated from patients or productions of conception.	Supportive.

(continued)

TABLE 11.3. (continued)

Disease	Epidemiology, Etiology, and/or Pathogenesis	Clinical Signs	Diagnosis	Initial Treatment (Alternate Rx in Parentheses)
3. Peripheral adenopathy a. Location varies with inoculation site				
1) Bacterial adenitis (associated with skin. Infection caused by group A streptococci or other pyogens)	Infection frequently follows skin trauma.	Streptococcal: Nodes are enlarged, tender, painful; sometimes no source apparent for lymphangitis; may see red streaks representing dilated painful lymphatics filled with exudate. May have overlying cellulitis. Axillary or inguinal involvement may progress to lymphedema with repeated attacks. Nonstreptococcal pyogenic infection may also be associated with lymphadenitis.	Can aspirate node and smear and culture if etiologic diagnosis is in doubt. Usually clinical characteristics are sufficient and the node does not require aspiration. Local cellulitis or skin lesions present should be aspirated, Gram stained, and cultured.	If streptococcal, use penicillin G. Some prefer antistaphylococcal penicillin to treat both staphylococci and streptococci. If other pyogens suspected, choose antibiotic on basis of predicted sensitivities.
2) Cat-scratch disease	Most patents have clearcut history of contact with cats; the local bite or scratch may or may not be obvious at the	1-3 weeks after cat contact, lesion appears at site, with regional node enlargement (usually axillary or epitrochlear).	Intradermal skin test (non-standardized and not generally available). Biopsy of node will show epithelioid granulomas,	If node purulent, may aspirate. Response to antibiotics is variable and seems

		time the node is inflamed. Etiology, currently thought to be *Bartonella* (formerly *Rochalimaea*) *henselae*.	Nodes may become fluctuant. Occasional patients have constitutional signs or a transient rash.	stellate abscesses, caseous necrosis, and giant cells. Silver stains demonstrate club-shaped organisms which are Gram-negative with Brown-Hopps stain. PCR may detect organisms in lesions.	more likely in the immunocompromised patient. Drugs used have included rifampin, ciprofloxacin, gentamicin and TMP-SMX.
3) Tularemia	Spread by (1) arthropod vectors-deerfly and ticks are especially important in the western U.S. in warm weather; (2) handling or eating infected animals (especially rabbits and muskrats) is a more common mode of spread in the eastern U.S., in the late winter hunting season; (3) airborne spread may occur, (4) waterborne epidemics have been reported.	Ulceroglandular tularemia: slightly painful papule that ulcerates, causing inflammation of regional nodes; these become tender, hot, and enlarged; accompanied by fever, myalgia, headache. Handling carcasses usually causes lesions on the hand with epitrochlear and axillary adenopathy. Arthropods may produce inoculation in different sites and resultant adenopathy may be cervical, inguinal, etc.	Culture (on cystine-containing medium) of blood, sputum, exudates, gastric washings. Serology is helpful but only after 10 days. Skin test may convert in 1st or 2nd week of illness (not readily available). Biopsy of nodes rarely needed, but if done, should be cultured and may show granulomas, micro-abscesses, caseous necrosis, and giant cells.	Streptomycin.

(continued)

TABLE 11.3. (continued)

Disease	Epidemiology, Etiology, and/or Pathogenesis	Clinical Signs	Diagnosis	Initial Treatment (Alternate Rx in Parentheses)
4) Plague	Disease of wild and domestic rodents transmitted to humans by rat flea. In U.S., endemic in the southwestern states. If pneumonia occurs, airborne spread may occur with potential for large serious epidemics with high mortality.	Fever and tender regional bubo, usually inguinal; can suppurate and drain spontaneously. If untreated, may progress to septicemia and to pneumonia. Bleeding tendency may produce ecchymoses.	Smear and culture blood, aspirate of bubo, and sputum; Giemsa stain better than Gram stain for visualization of Gram-negative "safety-pin" shaped organisms. Fluorescent stain. Serology helpful, but not positive until second week.	Streptomycin and tetracycline or chloramphenicol, but local resistance patterns may differ. Contacts of pneumonic cases should be treated with tetracycline, and patients with pneumonia require strictest respiratory isolation.
5) Rat-bite fever (S. minus)	Rat bite.	Incubation period 1–4 weeks, then bite flares when systemic illness begins. Regional nodes swell, become tender, firm and matted. May be accompanied by fever, rash, polyarthritis or arthralgia.	Dark field of bite, rash, or node aspirate will show organism; VDRL frequently positive. Specific serology may be performed.	Penicillin G or doxycycline.

LOCALIZED AND GENERALIZED LYMPHADENOPATHY

b. Usually axillary or epitrochlear			
1) Sporotrichosis	Organism lives on vegetation and in soil. Infection seen in people who work on farms or with plants, or who are exposed to contaminated vegetation.	Primary lesion: ulcerating nodule on extremities causing intermittent hard, red, suppurating nodules along lymph channels with regional adenopathy. No pain, fever or other constitutional symptoms.	Difficult to see organisms on smear, but can grow on Sabouraud's agar if nodule is aspirated.	Oral iodides for local disease.
2) Herpes zoster infection	Associated with stress, trauma, immunosuppression, and a depressed host resistance (e.g., in patients with lymphoma and other tumors). However, most cases occur without overt immunosuppressive states.	Clustered vesicles in unilateral segmental distribution; paresthesias, severe neuralgia, headache, and fever may accompany rash or precede it by several days. Regional adenitis is not very tender. (May disseminate).	Usually diagnosis can be made on basis of clinical findings alone. Stain scrapings from base of vesicle with Wright's or Giemsa's to demonstrate multinucleated giant cells and intranuclear inclusions. These findings are characteristic, but not pathognomonic for varicella-zoster virus. Culture is definitive.	Acyclovir or Famciclovir may shorten illness if given early.

(continued)

TABLE 11.3. (continued)

Disease	Epidemiology, Etiology, and/or Pathogenesis	Clinical Signs	Diagnosis	Initial Treatment (Alternate Rx in Parentheses)
3) Herpetic whitlow	Especially prevalent in nurses and dental personnel. Caused by *H. simplex* type 1. Rarely caused by *H. simplex* type 2, via inoculation from a genital lesion.	Swollen tender vesicular lesions on the pulp of the fingers; painful and tender regional adenopathy.	Vesicle can be unroofed, Gram stained, cultured for bacteria, and also stained for viral inclusions. Area of pulp inflammation should not be incised. Can be directly cultured for virus.	Acyclovir may be helpful.
c. Usually inguinal				
1) Primary syphilis	Venereal spread.	Painless genital chancre. Inguinal adenopathy that is painless, firm, freely movable, and nonsuppurating. Nodes may remain for months even though chancre heals in 2–6 weeks.	Serology helpful but may be negative early in primary disease.	Penicillin (doxycycline).
2) LGV	Usually venereal spread.	Primary painless genital papule/vesicle. Nodes: bilateral or unilateral inguinal adenopathy. Nodes may become	Organism may be isolated from pus in tissue culture, but this technique is not generally available. Serology	Doxycycline.

LOCALIZED AND GENERALIZED LYMPHADENOPATHY

| | | matted, multilocular, and suppurative, leading to multiple fistulae. Nodes tend to enlarge both above and below inguinal ligament. May produce rectal disease with diarrhea in females and homosexual males. Also seen at times are constitutional signs, including arthralgia and myalgias. | helpful. Biopsy characteristic: granulomas, microabscesses, caseous necrosis, and giant cells. | |
| 3) Chancroid | Venereal spread. | Chancres often multiple, painful, tender, and not indurated. Inguinal adenopathy painful and tender. Unilateral in 2/3. Untreated nodes may become matted and form a unilocular suppurative bubo. May rupture, causing a large single ulcer. | Smear and culture of node aspirate (specialized media). | Erythromycin (Azithromycin) (ciprofloxacin) (ceftriaxone). |

(continued)

TABLE 11.3. (continued)

Disease	Epidemiology, Etiology, and/or Pathogenesis	Clinical Signs	Diagnosis	Initial Treatment (Alternate Rx in Parentheses)
4) Granuloma inguinale	Some cases thought to be spread by venereal contact. Rare in U.S., seen mainly in tropics.	Chronic painless papule progressing to granulomatous tissue in inguinal region with subcutaneous swelling ("pseudo-bubo"). Node really not involved. Spreads by direct extension and destroys skin. Secondary bacterial infection may occur.	Stained impression smear from periphery of lesion shows "Donovan bodies" filling cytoplasm of large mononuclear cells. Culture in chick embryo yolk.	Doxycycline.
5) Genital herpes infection (Herpes simplex type II)	Venereal spread most common.	Painful vesicles on penis or in vagina and cervical area. May recur. Regional tender nodes are not uncommon.	Clinical appearance. Cervical smear shows atypical cells. Viral inclusions and multinucleate giant cells can be seen if lesion scraped and stained. Viral cultures positive for herpes.	Acyclovir helpful if given early in primary infection. It is less helpful in treatment of recurrences, although chronic suppressive therapy may prevent some recurrent attacks.

LOCALIZED AND GENERALIZED LYMPHADENOPATHY

B. Generalized lymphoadenopathy

1. Infectious mononucleosis	EBV infection, spread via oropharyngeal route. Virus may be present in pharynx months after infection occurs.	Most clinically significant cases occur in adolescents and young adults. Adenopathy may be generalized, with splenomegaly, supraorbital edema, and maculopapular rash.	Lymphocytosis with many atypical cells seen in peripheral smear. Significant anemia rare. Serology very helpful. Abnormal LFTs frequent. If serology negative for infectious mononucleosis, do serology for Hepatitis, HIV, toxoplasmosis, CMV, and possibly other viruses.	Supportive in most cases. Corticosteroids are helpful for laryngeal obstruction, extreme toxicity, hematologic and neurologic complications.
2. Rubella	Nasopharyngeal secretions are infectious. If disease occurs in pregnancy, products of conception are infectious and congenital rubella infection requires strict isolation.	Fever, faint pink macular rash; adenopathy; back of neck, especially along sternomastoid, around the mastoid, and in suboccipital locations. Adenopathy may be generalized. Nodes are small and only rarely tender; they may precede the rash.	Serology helpful.	Supportive.

(continued)

TABLE 11.3. *(continued)*

Disease	Epidemiology, Etiology, and/or Pathogenesis	Clinical Signs	Diagnosis	Initial Treatment (Alternate Rx in Parentheses)
3. CMV	Virus widespread in many body fluids, including blood, sputum, semen, breast milk, cervical secretions, and urine in healthy asymptomatic individuals. The fever-splenomegaly-lymphocytosis syndrome sometimes seen after open-heart surgery is often caused by this agent. Other patients at risk are recipients of whole blood, leukocytes, renal, heart and marrow transplants, and immunocompromised patients.	This agent causes a variety of clinical manifestations and frequently produces asymptomatic illness. Adenopathy is seen in both congenital and acquired disease and is particularly prominent in adult patients who present with an infectious mononucleosis-like syndrome. Fever and hepatitis are common, and serologic studies may convert late. The severe pneumonias seen with CMV usually occur in immunocompromised patients.	Culture urine, throat, and blood for CMV. Examine urine for inclusion bodies (rarely positive in acquired infections). Serology. Abnormal liver function tests. Peripheral smear: increased number of lymphocytes and many atypical lymphs, suggestive of infectious mononucleosis. Negative Monospot test and EBV serology.	Ganciclovir may be effective in immunocompromised patients.

4. Measles	Nasopharyngeal secretions of patients very infectious. Now occurs mainly in unimmunized population.	Fever, coryza, cough, Koplik's spots, red splatchy rash on face, then trunk. Lymphadenopathy may be generalized or predominate in occipital, mastoid, or posterior cervical regions.	Usually diagnosis is obvious clinically and laboratory studies need not be performed. Slight decrease in peripheral WBCs. Isolation of virus from urine and sputum. Serology helpful. Nodes show increased germinal follicles and multinucleate giant cells; same changes are seen in other organs, e.g., appendix.	After known exposure, gamma globulin is helpful in modifying illness if given early in incubation period.
5. Dengue	Arbovirus spread by Aedes mosquito in tropical and subtropical climates.	"Breakbone fever," with severe back and bone pain. Prodromal coryza, headache, myalgias, rash, arthralgias, occular soreness, scleral injection; adenopathy is posterior cervical, epitrochlear, and inguinal, and is usually nontender. Illness is diphasic.	Frequently WBCs very low. Virus isolation from blood. Serology helpful.	Symptomatic only.

(continued)

TABLE 11.3. (continued)

Disease	Epidemiology, Etiology, and/or Pathogenesis	Clinical Signs	Diagnosis	Initial Treatment (Alternate Rx in Parentheses)
6. Toxoplasmosis	Cat is definitive host; passes oocysts in feces, which are thought to infect many other mammals and birds. Some cases are caused by eating undercooked meat, especially pork and beef, which may contain cysts. No human-to-human transmission known except via placenta in congenital disease and in transplanted tissues. Severe infection seen in immunosuppressed hosts.	Infectious mononucleosis-like illness with fever, generalized lymphadenopathy, especially in cervical region. Nodes are firm, discreet, smooth, and may be painful and tender. They rarely suppurate. Rash present with lymphadenopathy not predominating. May present as FUO, myocarditis, pericarditis, encephalitis, pneumonitis, or hepatitis.	Serology is helpful. Lymph node biopsy findings are helpful even if no organisms are seen, but are not pathognomonic and sometimes resemble lymphoma. Agent may be isolated by inoculation of infectious tissue in mice. Wright's or Giemsa's stains of muscle, node, or CSF may demonstrate trophozoites or cysts. Polymerase chain reaction (PCR) may become useful in diagnosis.	Pyrimethamine and sulfadiazine (give folinic acid as well). (Most cases are self-limited and do not require therapy in immunocompetent patients.)

7. Tularemia	Spread by (1) arthropod vectors (deerfly and tick) are especially important in the western U.S. in warm weather; (2) handling or eating infected animals (especially rabbits and muskrats) is a more common mode of spread in the eastern U.S. in the late winter hunting season; (3) airborne spread may occur; (4) waterborne epidemics have been reported.	Ulceroglandular tularemia; slightly painful papule that ulcerates, causing inflammation of regional nodes; these become tender, hot and enlarged; accompanied by fever, myalgia, headache. Disease also has typhoidal or pulmonary form, and in these forms, adenopathy may be generalized.	Culture (on cystine-containing medium) of blood, sputum, exudates, gastric washings. Serology is helpful but only after 10 days. Skin test may convert in 1st or 2nd week of illness (not readily available). Biopsy of node rarely needed, but if done, should be cultured and may show granulomas, microabscesses, caseous necrosis, and giant cells.	Streptomycin.

(continued)

TABLE 11.3. (continued)

Disease	Epidemiology, Etiology, and/or Pathogenesis	Clinical Signs	Diagnosis	Initial Treatment (Alternate Rx in Parentheses)
8. Brucellosis	Direct contact with hogs, sheep, cattle, goats, and dogs. Also acquired by ingestion of contaminated milk or milk products.	Acute or chronic constitutional signs and fever associated with small, nontender cervical and axillary adenopathy and hepatosplenomegaly. Complications include osteomyelitis (usually spondylitis), endocarditis, and meningitis.	Culture blood, bone marrow and possibly liver. Be certain lab incubates under 10% CO_2 for at least 21 days. Serology helpful. If node or liver is biopsied, see granulomas, microabscesses, caseous necrosis, giant cells, calcification. These same changes may be seen in other organs as well, e.g., spleen, bone marrow.	Rifampin + doxycycline
9. Tuberculosis	Generalized adenopathy may be seen in the course of disseminated tuberculosis.	Usually evidence that tuberculous infection exists, particularly in the lungs. At times presents as an FUO with initially normal chest x-ray.	Chest x-ray, skin test. Smear and culture of sputum, culture of gastrics. Node biopsy may show giant cells, tubercles, caseous necrosis, fibrosis, calcification; lesion identical to those seen in other organs. Node must be cultured, as organisms are difficult to visualize. Bone-marrow and liver biopsies and culture are helpful diagnostic studies.	Isoniazid plus rifampin + ethambutol + pyrazinamide (corticosteroids useful for extreme toxicity).

10. Histoplasmosis	Exposure to dust or soil contaminated with excreta of birds, especially chickens, starlings, and bats.	In disseminated histoplasmosis may see generalized lymphadenopathy along with the hepatosplenomegaly.	Culture marrow, blood, sputum, and/or lymph nodes on specialized media. Smear of these specimens to look for organisms in macrophages.	Amphotericin B for disseminated disease.
11. Secondary syphilis	Primary syphilis is a venereally spread disease. Secondary syphilis occurs only if a primary case has not been adequately treated and generally occurs 2 weeks to 6 months after the primary.	Fever, diffuse rash, often including palms and soles, and generalized lymphadenopathy which is nontender often including pre and postauricular, occipital, and epitrochlear nodes. These may remain palpable for months after other signs of secondary syphilis have disappeared.	VDRL is as sensitive as FTA-ABS in secondary syphilis, but is not as specific.	Penicillin (doxycycline)
12. HIV	Generalized adenopathy may be seen during primary infection ("mono-like" illness). Generalized adenopathy may then return later in the course of the HIV infection as it becomes more advanced.	In primary infection, often accompanied by a diffuse, salmon-colored rash.	Serology.	No effective therapy for primary infection. For later manifestations of HIV infection, the benefit of anti-retroviral therapy appears to depend on presence of symptoms and the CD4 count. Exact indications for specific anti-HIV Rx continue to evolve and are presently inconclusive.

12

THE COMPROMISED HOST

Humans have evolved a complex system of defenses against microbial invasion. Infection frequently occurs when these defenses are compromised. In fact, the clinician can at times predict the type of infection a patient is likely to acquire, depending on which component of host resistance is disturbed. The best understood aspects of our ability to protect ourselves from infection are: (a) mechanical barriers of skin and mucous membranes, (b) bacterial inhibition by normal flora, (c) humoral immunity, or phagocytosis of invading microbes, a process that demands coordination between phagocytes, serum complement, and immunoglobulin, and (d) a system of cell-mediated immunity that attacks primarily intracellular pathogens by a complex interaction of T-lymphocytes, macrophages and cytokines.

DEFECTS IN HOST DEFENSE

Defects in any of the components of host resistance described above can result from underlying illness or from iatrogenic factors.

    Mechanical barriers. Barriers may be disrupted by urinary or IV catheterization, intubation, surgery, and burns and thereby allow microorganisms access to an otherwise sterile area, e.g., the urinary bladder, the lower respiratory tract, or the bloodstream.

Suppressed normal flora. Normal bacterial flora may be suppressed by antibiotic therapy or changed by severe underlying illness. For example, patients with chronic obstructive lung disease are more likely to be colonized by Gram-negative rods in their pharynx.

Impaired humoral immunity, or phagocytosis. Phagocytosis may be impaired if either serum factors such as specific antibody or heat-labile opsonins, or polymorphonuclear leukocyte (PML) function is altered. In this instance, patients are susceptible to pyogenic infection, especially with Gram-positive cocci, Gram-negative enteric bacilli and Haemophilus. Immunoglobulin deficiency may be congenital (e.g., Bruton's hypogammaglobulinemia) or acquired. Some acquired disease states associated with abnormal or insufficient immunoglobulins are burns, hypoproteinemic states (nephrotic syndrome, intestinal lymphangiectasia, etc.), multiple myeloma and chronic lymphocytic leukemia. Immunoglobulin levels may also be decreased by therapy with immunosuppressive drugs (e.g., cytotoxic agents) and certain antibiotics.

Opsonins other than specific antibody are also important in rendering bacteria more susceptible to phagocytosis. Such opsonins include the complement cascade, deficiencies of which may lessen a patient's ability to ward off infection. Defects of the early components of the complement cascade (C_1, C_2, C_4) do not always lead to increased susceptibility to infection, because C_3 may still be activated by the alternate (properdin) pathway. In sickle cell anemia, a disease in which pneumococcal infections of marked severity occur, a defect in the alternate pathway has been described. This pathway is especially important early in infection before specific antibody, which is necessary for triggering the "classical pathway," has been formed.

Complement deficiencies may be either congenital or acquired. It is possible that the reduction in complement components seen in diseases such as SLE (lupus) plays a significant role in the increased susceptibility to infection. Some patients with defects in the third and fifth components of complement have been plagued by multiple infections. Patients with defects in the late components of the complement system (C_5, C_6, C_7, C_8) have been reported with recurrent bouts of disseminated neisserial infections. Complement activities other than opsonization include kinin activation, viral neutralization, chemotaxis, cytolysis, neutrophil activation, and anaphylatoxin.

Opsonized bacteria must, of course, be ingested by adequately functioning PMLs. Therefore, PML dysfunction may be associated with serious infection. These cells may be decreased in number by toxins, irradiation, chemotherapeutic agents, or by tumor invading the marrow. In other situations the number of cells might be normal but their physiology may be severely disturbed, and abnormalities of (a) adherence to vascular endothelium, (b) chemotaxis, (c) ingestion, and (d) intracellular killing have all been documented. Examples of interference with each of these normal PML functions are listed in Table 12.1.

Defects of the cell-mediated immune system. This system is defective in a large group of disorders. A congenital prototype for this group is the DiGeorge syndrome of thymic hypoplasia. Acquired deficiencies in cell-mediated immunity are seen in the following:

Hodgkin's disease and other lymphomas
Sarcoidosis
Mucocutaneous candidiasis
Advanced tuberculosis
Lepromatous leprosy
Renal failure
SLE
Malnutrition
Metastatic carcinoma
Viral infection, especially measles, infectious mononucleosis, influenza, CMV
Intestinal lymphangiectasia
Pregnancy
AIDS

In addition, certain types of therapy may alter the cellular immune response, for example, irradiation and administration of corticosteroids and cytotoxic agents.

Rarely, some congenital syndromes are associated with a combined defect in cell-mediated immunity and immunoglobulin synthesis, e.g., (a) severe combined immunodeficiency (SCID), (b) Wiscott-Aldrich syndrome, and (c) ataxia-telangiectasis.

TABLE 12.1. ABNORMALITIES OF PML FUNCTION

Vascular adherence
  Leukocyte adhesion disorders
  Corticosteroids
  Salicylates
  Alcohol

Chemotaxis (either serum factors or cells or both may be responsible)
  Systemic lupus erythematosus (SLE)
  Cirrhosis
  Severe infection
  Hypophosphatemia (especially with hyperalimentation)
  Diabetes mellitus
  Neonatal state
  Chediak-Higashi syndrome
  Rheumatoid arthritis
  Daily administration of corticosteroids
  Hodgkin's disease
  Complement deficiency (C_3, C_5)
  Colchicine
  Renal disease
  Sarcoidosis
  Leprosy
  Burns
  Chronic alcoholism
  Hyper IgE
  "Lazy leukocyte" syndrome

Ingestion (either serum factors or cells or both may be responsible)
  Defective opsonization (decreased C_3, hypogammaglobulinemia of any cause, cirrhosis, low-birth-weight infants, SLE, AGN, sickle-cell anemia).
  Hyperosmolar states (e.g., hyperglycemia)
  Severe infection
  Hypophosphatemia (especially with hyperalimentation)
  Colchicine
  Cyclophosphamide
  Tetracycline
  Rheumatoid arthritis

(continued)

TABLE 12.1. *(continued)*

Intracellular killing
  Actin-myosin dysfunction
  Chloramphenicol
  Phenylbutazone
  Felty's syndrome
  Malakoplakia
  Burns
  CGD (Chronic granulomatous disease)
  Myeloperoxidase deficiency
  Severe infection
  Down's syndrome
  Craniospinal irradiation
  Hypophosphatemia
  Severe neutrophil G6PD deficiency
  Some patients with Job's syndrome

OPPORTUNISTIC PATHOGENS

When infected, patients with defects in host defenses may develop infections with agents that only rarely cause disease in normal individuals. This latter group of microbial agents, known as "opportunistic pathogens," is ubiquitous, and many of its members are present as part of the normal flora, for example, Candida. In addition some classical pathogens also infect compromised hosts, such as mycobacteria. The type of immune defect, i.e., humoral or cell-mediated, generally predicts which organisms are likely invaders (see Table 12. 2)

Patients with defects in humoral immunity (phagocytosis, complement, immunoglobulin) frequently develop infections with extracellular pyogenic bacteria such as pneumococci, staphylococci, pseudomonads, and more rarely with fungi such as Candida and Aspergillus. On the other hand, patients with inadequate cell-mediated immunity are more likely to become infected with intracellular bacteria (Listeria, Salmonella, mycobacteria), fungi such as Cryptococcus, parasites, and viruses in the herpes virus family (*H. simplex, Varicella-zoster* and CMV).

TABLE 12.2. TYPICAL PATHOGENS ASSOCIATED WITH HUMORAL OR T-CELL DEFECTS

	Humoral Defect (PMNs, Complement, Antibody)	T-Cell Defect
Bacteria	Pseudomonas Staphylococcus Enterobacteriaceae Streptococcus pneumoniae	Legionella Salmonella Listeria Nocardia Myocobacteria
Viruses	Hepatitis Enterovirus	CMV Herpes simplex Varicella-zoster
Fungi	Candida Aspergillus Mucormycosis	Cryptococcus Histoplasma
Parasites		Toxoplasma *P. carinii* Strongyloides Cryptosporidium Isospora Cyclospora Microsporidium

There are certain microorganisms that are associated with specific diseases. The specific relationships to be kept in mind are listed in Table 12.3.

To treat infections in the compromised host successfully, early recognition is imperative. This may not be easy since these patients frequently fail to respond to infections with the classical signs and symptoms, so that their infection may not be apparent until it has progressed considerably. For these reasons a physician working with these patients must maintain continued vigilance for infection. When infection is suspected in the compromised host, the initial studies are similar to those performed in the normal host. But, in addition, the opportunistic pathogens must also be considered, since specific therapy is available for many of these microbial agents.

TABLE 12.3. ASSOCIATION OF SPECIFIC MICROORGANISMS WITH PARTICULAR DISEASES OR CLINICAL STATES

Condition	Associated Organism
Alveolar proteinosis	Nocardia asteroides
Burns	S. aureus, streptococci, pseudomonads, Aspergillus, Candida, Phycomycetes, Herpes simplex
Chronic granulomatous disease	S. aureus, Gram-negative enteric bacilli (Catalase-negative organisms, e.g., pneumococci, streptococci, are not responsible for repeated infections in this group of patients)
Cirrhosis	Pneumococci and Gram-negative enteric rods
Cystic fibrosis	Pseudomonas, S. aureus
Diabetic ketoacidosis	Phycomycetes (nasopharyngeal)
Endocrinopathies (especially hypoparathyroidism)	Candida
GI Surgery	Gram-negative enteric aerobes, Bacteroides, Candida, bowel streptococci
Hemolytic states	Salmonella
Lymphoma	Cryptococcus, varicella-zoster, P. carinii
Hypochlorhydric states	M. tuberculosis, Salmonella
Leukemia	Pseudomonas, other Gram-negative rods, Aspergillus, Phycomycetes (pulmonary), P. carinii

(continued)

TABLE 12.3. (continued)

Multiple myeloma	Pneumococcus and other pyogenic bacteria
Nephrotic syndrome	Pneumococcus
Neutropenia	Pseudomonas, other Gram-negative rods
Sickle cell disease	Salmonella, Pneumococcus, Mycoplasma
Splenectomy	Pneumococcus. H. influenzae
Transplant recipient receiving immunosuppressives	P. carinii, CMV, Aspergillus, Candida albicans, Toxoplasma
AIDS	P. carinii, Toxoplasma, TB, Cryptococcus (see chapter on AIDS)

PULMONARY INFILTRATE IN THE COMPROMISED HOST

The approach to a common problem confronting the compromised host, namely, the combination of fever and pulmonary infiltrate, is now illustrated. In this situation, the clinician must be aware of the possible causes of this syndrome. The four most likely etiologies are:

1. Bacterial infection (pneumococci, Gram-negative rods, staphylococci, Legionella)
2. Opportunistic infections (fungi, *P. carinii*, viruses, mycobacteria, Toxoplasma)
3. Underlying disease (e.g., lymphoma, leukemia)
4. Reactions to drugs (e.g., cytoxan, busulphan, bleomycin, methotrexate)

COMPROMISED HOST

If a patient is critically ill, one must choose techniques that can rapidly establish the diagnosis. Unfortunately, examination of the sputum is not always conclusive, and therefore one may need to proceed quickly to (a) bronchoscopy to obtain brush biopsies, bronchial washings, and/or transbronchial biopsies, or (b) lung biopsies (either percutaneously or by limited thoracotomy).

All specimens obtained in the compromised host, whether sputum, urine, blood, other body fluids, or biopsies, should be handled to assure recovery and identification of opportunistic pathogens, as well as of the more routine microbial invaders. This requires a coordinated approach by the clinician, pathologist, and microbiologist. As usual, all specimens should be sent to the microbiology laboratory to be stained and cultured for bacteria, fungi, parasites, and suspected viruses. Immunofluorescent stains and recently developed molecular biologic techniques such as polymerase chain reaction (PCR) are particularly helpful when available.

Another portion of the specimen is sent to pathology, where immediate stains may be performed. A lung biopsy specimen, for example, can be immediately stained with a silver preparation, looking for fungi or *P. carinii*. Most viral inclusions are demonstrable by Giemsa staining, although immunofluorescent and immunoperoxidase stains are sometimes helpful. Fungi may be demonstrated by Gram, Gomori, and PAS stains, but mucicarmine is especially valuable in identifying Cryptococci. Acid-fast stains may help diagnose Nocardia or mycobacterial infection. Toxoplasma are best identified with Wright's or a Giemsa stain. Legionnaire's agent may be identified by silver and fluorescent antibody staining. An irrevocable error that is made with distressing frequency is the failure to send biopsy specimens for culture before they are fixed in formalin. If proper handling is in doubt (check with the microbiologist) send tissue in a dry sterile container and fluid in a capped syringe.

GENERAL THERAPEUTIC GUIDELINES

Treatment of infection in the compromised host should be directed against the specific infecting pathogen when possible. At times presumptive therapy based on the most likely possibilities must be started as soon as appropriate studies have been obtained. Unfortunately, it is sometimes impossible to obtain needed specimens for smear or culture. For example, a leukemic patient with severe thrombocytopenia who has a progressive pulmonary infiltrate, severe hypoxia, and no sputum production, cannot have transtracheal aspiration, bronchoscopy, or lung biopsy procedures performed without hazard. Occasionally, biopsy may be done in such patients after platelet transfusions. When tissue is not obtainable in critically ill patients who have compromised host defenses, a therapeutic regimen including treatment for *P. carinii* and fungi as well as antibiotics for the more common bacterial and nonbacterial pulmonary pathogens may be justified. Thus in this dire situation, a representative regimen might contain trimethoprim-sulfamethoxazole, amphotericin B, gentamicin, erythromycin and a cephalosporin.

Although appropriate antimicrobial therapy is crucial, the infection may continue uncontrolled unless the underlying compromising factors can be eliminated. Thus neutrophil transfusions and the various leukocyte stimulating factors could be considered in the treatment of infection in patients with severe granulocytopenia.

The iatrogenic causes of diminished host resistance should also be eliminated. One should attempt to either discontinue or reduce the dose of corticosteroid or cytotoxic therapy when possible, although the steroid dose for patients receiving long-term corticosteroid therapy must be maximized temporarily during times of stress, to avoid adrenal insufficiency. In some instances of serious infection in renal transplant recipients, immunosuppressive therapy might be discontinued even at the expense of allowing the transplant to be rejected, in order to permit an adequate host response to infection. On the other hand, institution or maintenance of chemotherapy to induce remission in a leukemic patient may offer the only hope of cure of the infection. These decisions are complex and must be individualized for each patient.

PREVENTIVE MEASURES

Preventive measures are extremely important when caring for these patients. Meticulous attention must be given to such simple procedures as:

(1) appropriate hand washing,
(2) correct urinary and IV catheter insertion and care,

(3) avoidance of unnecessary antibiotics,
(4) appropriate isolation techniques, when indicated
(5) cleaning of respiratory therapy equipment,
(6) assistance from a hospital infection control officer to help decrease the incidence of infection.

More specific protective methods include the use of certain vaccines (e.g., influenza and pneumococcal vaccine) and the use of antisera such as ZIG (zoster immune globulin). At no time, however, should an immunocompromised individual receive live vaccines. Laminar flow systems, routine prophylactic antibiotics and various elaborate isolation rituals all have disappointingly limited effectiveness, and the most helpful prophylactic measures are one through six listed.

TABLE 12.4. DIAGNOSTIC CHART: INFECTION IN THE COMPROMISED HOST—SELECTED ETIOLOGIES*

Disease	Predisposition	Clinical	Diagnosis	Initial Treatment
A. Mycotic infection	In general, patients who have deficient host defenses are particularly susceptible to the fungal infections outlined below. Especially susceptible are patients with altered cellular immunity and those with prior antibiotic, corticosteroid, or immunosuppressive therapy.		Sputum culture of Candida and Aspergillus may represent normal flora or contaminants. Phycomycetes are common molds that are not infrequent laboratory contaminants.	
1. Candidiasis	Most frequent opportunist of all the fungi. Seen with cancer, surgery (especially of the GI tract), IV catheters, burns, blood dyscrasias, hyperalimentation, antibiotic use, and corticosteroid and cytotoxic drug administration.	Fungemia, pyelonephritis, endophthalmitis, skin lesions, widespread tissue invasion. Pneumonia may occur via bloodstream dissemination or aspiration.	Culture is of help only if from otherwise sterile tissue. The presence of Candida in expectorated sputum does not prove the etiology of a lower respiratory tract infection, since the organism may contaminate the upper airway. Lung biopsy should be done for morphology, staining and culture. Culture blood and urine. Buffy coat smear of blood. Appearance of	Amphotericin B; 5-fluorocytosine may be added if organism shown to be sensitive. Flucytosine is an alternative.

		endophthalmitis very suggestive. Absence of organisms in urine is fairly strong evidence against disseminated candidiasis.	
2. Cryptococcosis	AIDS, lymphoproliferative diseases (particularly Hodgkin's disease), diabetes, transplant recipients or other patients receiving corticosteroids or cytotoxic agents.	Disseminated disease frequently presents as meningitis. At times only pulmonary or other metastatic infection is seen.	Culture of blood, sputum, CSF, urine biopsy and stain of tissue. India ink prep on CSF, sputum, urine. CRAG.	Amphotericin B and 5-fluorocytosine; Flucytosine.
3. Invasive aspergillosis	Immunosuppressed patients, especially those with acute leukemia. Also immunosuppressed transplant recipients.	Chest x-ray may resemble bacterial pneumonia or lung abscess, if pulmonary involvement present. Hematogenous dissemination may occur.	Culture most reliable only from lung tissue but if patient's at risk, a nasal or sputum culture correlates well with Aspergillus pneumonia. The upper airway may be contaminated with the organism; conversely, sputum culture may be falsely negative despite pneumonia. Biopsy is characteristic (shows branching septate hyphae). Blood cultures are usually negative.	Amphotericin B.

(continued)

274   DIFFERENTIAL DIAGNOSIS OF INFECTIOUS DISEASES

TABLE 12.4. *(continued)*

Disease	Predisposition	Clinical	Diagnosis	Initial Treatment
4. Phycomycosis	Acidosis (especially diabetic), lymphoma/leukemia, and malnutrition all predispose.	Acidosis associated with rhinocerebral infection with orbital cellulitis, sinusitis, bloody nasal discharge, necrotic turbinates, and CNS extension. Leukemia/lymphoma especially associated with pneumonia. Malnutrition associated with GI infection causing problems ranging from gastroenteritis with bloody stool to perforation.	Scrapings with KOH preparation or PAS stain helpful. Cultures usually negative. Accessible lesions should be biopsied and stained to show characteristic wide nonseptate hyphae with evidence of tissue and vascular invasion.	Usually need both amphotericin B and radical debridement. Reverse acidosis if present.
B. Bacterial infection				
1. Nocardiosis	Corticosteroid and immunosuppressive therapy, malignancy, alveolar proteinosis.	Chest x-ray may resemble TB, bacterial pneumonia, or multiple lung abscesses. May spread to CNS or bone.	Gram stain shows delicate Gram-positive branching rods that are acid-fast if acid-fast staining is performed with weak decolorization.	Sulfonamides are mainstay of therapy, but trimethoprim-sulfamethoxazole or minocycline may be useful.

		Bacterial and fungal cultures should be performed, but may take several days or weeks to grow. The organism grows aerobically. Tissue should be stained with gram, acid-fast, and silver.
2. Listeriosis	Immunocompromised patients, especially with lymphoma, or receiving corticosteroids or cytotoxic therapy.	Fever, bacteremia, meningitis.	Gram stain of CSF is ⊕ in only 50%. Culture blood and CSF.	Ampicillin usually satisfactory, but sensitivities variable.
C. Parasitic infection				
1. *P. carinii*	Immunosuppressed patients, especially with AIDS, leukemia/lymphoma, and/or those receiving corticosteroids.	Pneumonia, diffuse patchy infiltrates, interstitial pattern, or multiple nodules. Severe progressive dyspnea. Frequently seen in association with CMV infection of the lung.	Characteristic chest x-ray and progressive hypoxia. Bronchial lavage as sensitive as transbronchial biopsy in experienced hands. PCR helpful when available.	Trimethoprim-sulfamethoxazole.

(continued)

COMPROMISED HOST

TABLE 12.4. *(continued)*

Disease	Predisposition	Clinical	Diagnosis	Initial Treatment
2. Toxoplasmosis	Immunosuppressed patients, especially with AIDS.	Disseminated disease may involve the CNS, heart, liver, and lungs. In AIDS see multiple brain abscesses.	Serology. Biopsy of involved tissues with appropriate stains such as Giemsa or Wright for trophozoites or PAS for cysts. Lymph node and muscle are good sources for biopsy. May attempt culture of the organisms in mice. PCR may become useful.	Pyrimethamine and sulfadiazine.
3. Strongyloides hyperinfection syndrome	Intestinal strongyloidiasis (usually asymptomatic) plus immunosuppression.	Fever, confusion, diffuse pulmonary infiltrates.	See larvae in sputum. Eosinophilia uncommon.	Treat for strongyloides with thiabendazole. Also, many patients have associated Gram-negative bacteremia or meningitis.
D. Viral infections				
1. Varicella-zoster infection	Immunosuppressed patients, especially those with lymphoma or leukemia.	Pneumonia, at times with hemorrhage; disseminated renal or visceral disease; severe prolonged skin eruptions.	Giemsa or Wright's stains of scrapings from base of fresh vesicle (Tzanck smear) show multinucleated giant cells and nuclear inclusions in	Acyclovir.

2. CMV infection	Malignancy, especially leukemia/lymphoma; administration of corticosteroids or cytotoxic drugs, especially after renal and marrow transplants.	Interstitial pneumonia; hepatitis, colitis.	both varicella-zoster and *H. simplex* infection. Sputum may show typical intranuclear inclusions. Viral isolation can be attempted from infected material. Antigen may be detected in vesicles by fluorescent antibody techniques. Serology.	
			Urine and throat viral cultures; serology. Inclusion bodies in nucleus and cytoplasm of cells in urine should be looked for, but are rarely seen in adults with acquired diseases. Inclusion bodies may be seen in bronchial washings of patients with pneumonia. Biopsy of lung or liver may show characteristic cytomegalic cells.	Ganciclovir

(continued)

TABLE 12.4. (continued)

Disease	Predisposition	Clinical	Diagnosis	Initial Treatment
3. Herpes simplex infection	Immunosuppression, especially for renal transplant recipients; Hodgkin's disease; Wiscott-Aldrich syndrome; burns; atopic eczema.	Severe localized disease or disseminated infection.	Isolation in tissue culture from vesicle fluid or involved tissue; serology; characteristic histologic changes in tissue, although in brain tissue, similar changes may result from varicella-zoster and measles viruses. Tzanck smear of skin lesions shows multinucleated giant cells and intranuclear inclusions, indistinguishable from changes seen in varicella-zoster infection.	Acyclovir

*Only diseases produced by opportunistic pathogens are discussed. Common bacteria are still the most frequent cause of infection in the compromised host, but are omitted here so that these rarer and often treatable infections can be emphasized.

13

AIDS

Acquired Immunodeficiency Syndrome (AIDS) is the result of infection with the human immunodeficiency virus (HIV) that has reached an advanced stage.

HIV is spread by direct inoculation of infected blood or body fluids. The inoculation may occur in mucous membranes or broken skin. Thus, the groups at greatest risk are intravenous drug abusers who share needles and/or sexual contacts of infected patients. A small proportion of patients acquires the virus via blood transfusion and exposure to contaminated articles like toothbrushes and razors.

After an incubation period of two to four weeks, most patients have an early illness that resembles infectious mononucleosis. Fever, myalgias, sore throat and lymphadenopathy are common; many patients have a maculopapular rash which has a characteristic salmon color and may involve the palms and soles. On occasion the eruption is urticarial or vesicular. Ulcerations may involve mucocutaneous areas and thus suggest secondary syphilis. Antibodies develop within a few weeks of this initial illness, although the P24 antigen is detectable in serum and spinal fluid as early as 24 hours after the acute illness begins. (Polymerase chain reaction (PCR) has also detected HIV nucleic acid in blood mononuclear cells and in serum early in infection.)

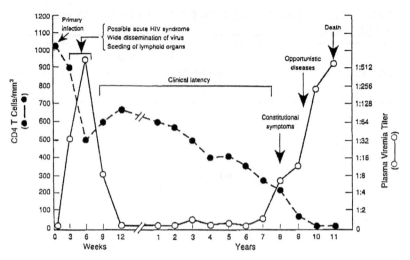

Figure 13.1. Typical course of HIV infection. During the early period after primary infection there is widespread dissemination of virus and a sharp decrease in the number of CD4 T cells in peripheral blood. An immune response to HIV ensues, with a decrease in detectable viremia followed by a prolonged period of clinical latency. The CD4 T-cell count continues to decrease during the following years, until it reaches a critical level below which there is a substantial risk of opportunistic diseases. Pantaleo G, Graziosi C, Fauci AS. The Immunopathogenesis of Human Immunodeficiency Virus Infection. *N. Engl. J. Med.* 328:327–335, 1993.

Clinical features which distinguish acute HIV infection from EB virus mononucleosis are the slow onset and more dramatic exudative pharyngotonsillitis seen with EB viral infection.

Figure 13.1 shows the course of HIV infection, indicating the CD4 count and viral titers during primary infection, latency and clinical deterioration. As the CD4 cell count declines, patients become susceptible to an increasing array of opportunistic infections and neoplasms. Thus, patients with CD4 counts in the 200 to 500 range develop tuberculosis, oroesophageal candidiasis and Kaposi's sarcoma. When the CD4 count drops below 200, patients develop *Pneumocystis carinii* pneumonia, cryptococcal infection and dementia, and CD4 counts below 50 are associated with toxoplasmosis, cytomegalovirus infection, and *Mycobacterium avium* complex (MAC). Death often ensues at this low level of immunity.

TABLE 13.1. CDC CLASSIFICATION SYSTEM FOR HIV INFECTION

CD4 Count	Clinical Category (see text)		
	A	B	C
1. 500/ml	A1	B1	C1[a]
2. 200–499/ml	A2	B2	C2[a]
3. < 200/ml	A3[a]	B3[a]	C3[a]

[a] = AIDS.
Adapted from *MMWR,* Vol 41, No. RR-17, Dec 18, 1992.

Classification systems for HIV infection use as parameters both the patient's clinical status and the number or percentage of CD4 cells, since the latter subgroup of lymphocytes declines with advancing disease and correlates well with the infectious and neoplastic complications of HIV infection.

The CDC staging system (Table 13.1) categorizes a patient's clinical status as Category A, B, or C. Category A includes patients with acute (primary) HIV infection, asymptomatic HIV infection or persistent generalized lymphadenopathy. Category B comprises symptomatic conditions such as bacillary angiomatosis, oropharyngeal or vulvovaginal candidiasis, hairy leukoplakia, idiopathic thrombocytopenic purpura and others. Category C includes the clinical conditions that are part of the Surveillance Case definition; these are listed in Table 13.2. The CDC system further assigns patients to one of three CD4 T lymphocyte categories: greater than 500 cells/mm^3, 200 to 499 cells/mm^3, and fewer than 200 cells/mm^3. All patients in clinical Category C and all patients with fewer than 200 CD4 cells (i.e., A3, B3, C1, C2, C3) are reportable as AIDS cases in the United States.

Diagnosis and management are particularly difficult in this syndrome, not only because many of the infections relapse and are difficult to treat, but also because patients simultaneously may have more than one infecting microorganism. Also, medical side effects of therapy are common and may resemble signs of infec-

TABLE 13.2. CONDITIONS INCLUDED IN THE 1993 AIDS SURVEILLANCE CASE DEFINITION

Candidiasis of bronchi, trachea, or lungs

Candidiasis, esophageal

Cervical cancer, invasive

Coccidioidomycosis, disseminated or extrapulmonary

Cryptococcosis, extrapulmonary

Cryptosporidiosis, chronic, intestinal (>1 month's duration)

Cytomegalovirus retinitis (with loss of vision)

Encephalopathy, HIV-related

Herpes simplex: chronic ulcer(s) (>1 month's duration); or bronchitis, pneumonitis, or esophagitis

Histoplasmosis, disseminated or extrapulmonary

Isosporiasis, chronic intestinal (>1 month's duration)

Kaposi's sarcoma

Lymphoma, Burkitt's (or equivalent term)

Lymphoma, immunoblastic (or equivalent term)

Lymphoma, primary, of brain

Mycobacterium avium complex or *M. kansasii,* disseminated or extrapulmonary

Mycobacterium tuberculosis, any site (pulmonary or extrapulmonary)

Mycobacterium, other species or unidentified species, disseminated or extrapulmonary

Pneumocystis carinii pneumonia

Pneumonia, recurrent

Progressive multifocal leukoencephalopathy

Salmonella septicemia, recurrent

Toxoplasmosis of brain

Wasting syndrome due to HIV

Adapted from *MMWR*, Vol 41, No. RR-17, Dec 18, 1992.

tion. Thus, rash may develop as a consequence of therapy with TMP-SMX, clindamycin, Fluconazole or pyrimethamine- sulfadiazine. Liver function test abnormalities may complicate therapy with TMP-SMX, pentamidine, clindamycin, ketoconazole, pyrimethamine-sulfadiazine, INH, rifampin, PZA, and Didanosine (ddI). Pancreatitis may develop from ddI, Zalcitabine (ddC), Stavudine (d4T) and pentamidine. Diarrhea, another common symptom, may be a side effect of therapy with clindamycin, fluconazole, ddI, and ciprofloxacin. Peripheral neuropathy can complicate treatment with ddC, ddI and d4T. Thus, symptoms may result from the infecting agent, from medication, or both.

A variety of infectious syndromes is seen in AIDS (Table 13.3). Infectious complications in AIDS result from HIV infection *per se* or from opportunistic infection complicating the HIV- induced immune deficiency. Thus, therapy is directed at both the HIV virus (antiretroviral therapy) and the individual opportunistic pathogens. Antiretroviral therapy delays disease progression and appears to prolong survival in advanced disease. At the present writing, antiretroviral therapy is administered to patients with CD4 counts below 500 if they are symptomatic or below 200 regardless of symptoms. It is also administered for specific clinical complications, i.e., dementia, peripheral neuropathy, myelopathy, immune thrombocytopenia, psoriasis, lymphocytic interstitial pneumonia (LIP), and to prevent neonatal infection by administration to HIV + mothers during pregnancy and then to the newborn. *Controversial* indications include HIV + patients with CD4 counts above 200 but no symptoms, and prophylactic administration to health care workers following occupational exposure. Zidovudine (AZT or ZDV) is the antiretroviral therapy of choice. When Zidovudine is not tolerated or not effective, other agents can be substituted or added, i.e., Didanosine (ddI) or Zalcitabine (ddC) or Stavudine (d4T).

MAJOR CLINICAL SYNDROMES

Constitutional signs and symptoms, predominantly fever and weight loss, may indicate generalized infection due to M. Avium complex (MAC), *M. tuberculosis* (MTB), Histoplasma or Cryptococcus. Cultures should be performed of blood, sputum, and

TABLE 13.3. AIDS: MAJOR INFECTIOUS COMPLICATIONS BY SYSTEM

I. Constitutional syndromes
   A. MAC, TB, histoplasmosis, bacteremia, cryptococcosis, tumor

II. Gastrointestinal
   A. Oral—Candida, *H. simplex* (HSV), cytomegalovirus (CMV), Histoplasmosis, EBV, human papillomavirus (HPV), bacterial infection
   B. Esophageal—Candida, CMV, HSV, idiopathic
   C. Diarrhea—Cryptosporidium, Isospora, Microsporidium Cyanobacteria, MAC, Salmonella, *C. difficile,* CMV, Shigella, Campylobacter, Giardia, amebae, HSV, Strongyloides
   D. Hepatobiliary—Cryptosporidium, CMV, MAC, Candida, Bartonella

III. Neurologic
   A. Meningoencephalitis—Toxoplasma (toxo), Crypto, TB, progressive multifocal leukoencephalopathy, HIV, syphilis, bacteria
   B. Myelitis—HIV, Varicella-Zoster (V-Z), HSV, toxo, CMV, TB, syphilis, HTLV-1, idiopathic
   C. Cranial neuropathy
   D. Peripheral neuropathy

IV. Skin
   A. Nodules—Bartonella, Molluscum, fungi, mycobacteria
   B. Vesicles/pustules—V-Z, staphylococcus, HSV, fungi, AFB
   C. Hyperkeratotic crusting—*S. scabei*
   D. Ulceration—HSV, AFB, fungi

V. Pulmonary
   A. *P. carinii* (PCP), TB, MAC, Histo, cocci, crypto, bacteria, CMV, V-Z

VI. Cardiac
   A. Myocarditis—non-specific, viruses, crypto, toxo, TB
   B. Endocarditis—staphylococcus, marantic
   C. Pericarditis—TB, MAC, crypto

VII. Myositis—staphylococcus

VIII. Sinusitis—*H. influenzae*, pneumococcus, Pseudomonas

IX. Eye
   A. Retinitis—CMV, toxo, idiopathic
   B. Endophthalmitis—candida
   C. Optic neuritis—syphilis, crypto

skin lesions. Also, bacteremias may complicate pneumonia, gastrointestinal infection, IV catheter infection or be "primary." In addition, some patients may develop a wasting illness due to Kaposi's sarcoma or nonHodgkin's lymphoma.

The entire gastrointestinal tract may be infected. Beginning with the mouth, oral lesions range from the pseudomembranes seen in candidiasis to the ulcerations of herpes simplex virus (HSV), cytomegalovirus (CMV) and Histoplasma. Hairy leukoplakia is attributed to Epstein-Barr virus, and nonspecific gingivitis is common. Esophagitis most frequently results from candidiasis and is frequently treated empirically for this pathogen. However, when this treatment fails, other organisms, particularly CMV and herpes, should be suspected and biopsy performed.

Enterocolitis may result from a variety of organisms, including bacteria, viruses, fungi, parasites, and mycobacteria. The specific syndromes are not diagnostic, and diagnosis depends on stains and culture of stool and biopsy of intestinal mucosa. In addition to routine bacterial stool cultures and stains for ova and parasites, additional tests on stool and biopsy material should include an assay for *C. difficile* toxin, Gram stain for microsporidium, and acid-fast stain for Cryptosporidium, Isospora, MAC, TB, and Cyanobacteria. Pseudoappendicitis in AIDS may be due to the traditional causes of this entity, i.e. Salmonella, Yersinia and Campylobacter, and also to processes characteristic of the AIDS patient, i.e. bacterial typhlitis, cecal CMV, and tuberculosis.

Hepatobiliary syndromes present as papillary stenosis, cholangitis or cholecystitis, and result from infection due to organisms such as CMV, Cryptosporidium, Microsporidium, MAC, and Candida. In addition, the entity of peliosis hepatis is currently attributed to infection with Bartonella (formerly Rochalimaea).

The most common neurologic syndrome in AIDS is the AIDS dementia complex, a chronic encephalitis probably caused by the HIV virus itself. It is nonspecific and is a diagnosis of exclusion. The HIV virus also may cause an acute meningitis during the initial infectious mono-like syndrome. Some patients have multiple relapses of this acute meningitis. Another common meningoencephalitis, especially in later stages of immunodeficiency, is caused by cryptococcal infection. Meningoencephalitis can also be caused by tuberculosis, HIV, varicella-zoster, syphilis, and multiple bacterial pathogens. Toxoplasmal infection produces focal or diffuse disease, with characteristic multiple ring-enhancing lesions on CT or MRI. Direct infection of the spinal cord (myelitis) may complicate infection due to a variety of viruses (HIV, *Varicella-zoster, Herpes simplex*, and CMV) and Toxoplasma. A related syndrome entitled spastic paraparesis is attributed to HTLV-1. In addition, a variety of peripheral neuropathies are described, due to HIV itself, herpes zoster, CMV, and autoimmune vascular processes. Unfortunately, many drugs used in the treatment of AIDS may cause peripheral neuropathy, as noted above. In addition, an autonomic neuropathy occurs commonly in advanced disease. In these neurologic infections, it is important to establish a diagnosis using specific tests, such as culture and antigen determination, since many HIV-positive patients have a nonspecific CSF pleocytosis and protein elevation, even while they are asymptomatic.

Dermatologic manifestations are legion. Bacillary angiomatosis produces vascular nodules that respond to therapy with erythromycin. Papular eruptions may also be seen with cutaneous or disseminated fungal infection, mycobacterial infection and molluscum contagiosum. Painful vesicles may indicate zoster, and pustules are frequently a result of staphylococcal infection. Herpes simplex virus may cause a typical vesicular eruption which progresses to ulceration and widespread necrosis. Ulcerations are also seen in mycobacterial and fungal infection. Hyperkeratotic lesions with crusting may indicate scabies.

Pneumonia is common in AIDS. Bacterial infection due to routine pathogens like pneumococcus and Haemophilus may occur and resemble the disease seen in immunocompetent patients. On the other hand, diffuse infiltrates are frequently seen and, while usually due to *Pneumocystis carinii* pneumonia, may also indicate infection due to Histoplasma, Coccidioides and Cryptococcus. In advanced disease, MAC may also produce diffuse interstitial infiltrates. Tuberculosis produces characteristic changes of TB in early HIV infection, but, in the advanced stages of AIDS, tuberculous infection behaves atypically and may cause adenopathy, abscess formation and diffuse or localized infiltrates. However, pneumocystis is common enough so that most clinicians treat empirically for this pathogen in the presence of diffuse interstitial infiltrates and a CD4 count lower than 200/mm^3.

Cardiac involvement in AIDS takes the form of myocarditis (nonspecific, or specific due to viruses, Cryptococcus, Toxoplasma and tuberculosis), endocarditis, and pericarditis due to mycobacterial or fungal infection.

Sinusitis may be severe and, in the presence of low numbers of CD4 cells, often affects multiple sinuses, producing chronic disease. Both bacteria and fungi may be etiologic.

Ophthalmologic complications include retinitis which may be nonspecific, may be due to cytomegalovirus in advanced disease, and, rarely, complicates Toxoplasma infection. Endophthalmitis may complicate bacteremia or fungemia, and optic neuritis complicates syphilis and cryptococcal meningitis.

Management of these patients requires not only recognition and treatment of specific infections, but also prophylaxis of infection. Thus, primary prophylaxis (before the first episode of infection) is recommended for *P. carinii*, TB, MAC and toxoplasmosis. Secondary prophylaxis, or suppressive therapy after treatment for acute infection is recommended for pneumocystosis, toxoplasmosis, cryptococcosis, histoplasmosis, coccidioidomycosis, Salmonella bacteremia, and cytomegaloviral infection, and may be indicated for selected patients with frequent severe recurrences of candidiasis and mucocutaneous herpes. Immunizations should be maintained with the vaccines for pneumococcus, influenza, hepatitis B and *Haemophilus influenzae*; finally, preventive dentistry may prevent some of the oral infectious complications such as gingivitis.

TABLE 13.4. DIAGNOSTIC CHART: AIDS–INFECTIOUS COMPLICATIONS

Syndrome	Etiology	Clinical	Diagnosis	Treatment
Constitutional				
	MAC	Systemic (fever, wt. loss) diarrhea, malabsorption, biliary obstruction.	Blood culture and sensitivity (not culture from stool, urine or sputum).	Clarithromycin + ethambutol ± rifampin ± ciprofloxacin Primary prophylaxis (<75 CD4 cells): Rifabutin.
	MTB	Pulmonary disease, adenopathy.	Culture and sensitivity of blood, sputum, marrow.	Prophylaxis for PPD 5 mm, or contact: INH. INH + rifampin + ethambutol + pyrazinamide as initial R. If MDR-TB strongly suspected treat pending culture results with Amikocin, ofloxacin, ETH and PZA + possibly additional drugs. For prophylaxis of MDR-TB, use PZA + ofloxacin. For prophylaxis of INH-resistant organisms: RIF + ETH
	Histoplasmosis	"Disseminated histoplasmosis."—Resp. symptoms in ½. Mucocutaneous ulcers, adenopathy, hepatosplenomegaly.	Culture and sensitivity of sputum, blood. Biopsy of ulcers, marrow.	Amphotericin B. Secondary prophylaxis: itraconazole.

	Bacteremia.	Ass'd with pneumonia (Pneumococcus, *H. influenzae*), G-I disease (Salmonella, Shigella, Campylobacter), with catheters (staph) and "primary" (Pseudomonas, *E. coli*, Klebsiella, Rochalimea).	Culture.	According to sensitivity.
	Cryptococcosis.	Skin lesions may mimic molluscum contagiosum.	Culture and sensitivity, CRAG.	Amphotericin B. Fluconazole. Secondary prophylaxis: Fluconazole.
	Tumor.	Kaposi's, Non-Hodgkins lymphoma.	Biopsy.	
G-I: Oral				
	Candida.	Pseudomembranes, erythema, chelitis.	KOH prep, culture and sensitivity.	Nystatin. Ketoconazole. Fluconazole. Secondary prophylaxis with Fluconazole.
	HSV.	Ulcerations on palate or gingiva.	Immunofluorescence. Tzanck smear.	Acyclovir. Secondary prophylaxis-acyclovir.
	CMV.	Ulcerations.	Biopsy.	Ganciclovir.
	Histoplasma.	Single lesion, ulcerations.	Biopsy, culture and sensitivity.	Amphotericin B. Secondary prophylaxis: itraconazole.

(continued)

TABLE 13.4. (continued)

Syndrome	Etiology	Clinical	Diagnosis	Treatment
G-I: Oral				
	EBV.	Hairy leukoplakia—corrugated white patches on lateral tongue.	Biopsy.	Acyclovir.
	HPV.	Warts.	Clinical.	Excision (surgical or laser).
	Bacterial infection.	Gingivitis, periodontitis—pain, bleeding, halitosis, ulcers, erythema.	Clinical.	Debridement, topical antiseptic. Amoxicillin-clavulanate.
G-I: Esophagitis				
	Candida.	Dysphagia. Suspect when oral thrush present.	Barium swallow; biopsy of plaques.	Ketoconazole, Fluconazole. Secondary prophylaxis-Fluconazole.
	CMV.	Odynophagia, suspect when Rx for Candida fails.	Endoscopy shows large shallow ulcers, biopsy.	Ganciclovir (relapse common).
	Herpes simplex.	Odynophagia—suspect when Rx for Candida fails.	Endoscopy shows small deep ulcers; biopsy.	Acyclovir. Secondary prophylaxis—acyclovir.
	Idopathic.	Odynophagia.	Other studies ⊖, ulcers.	Steroids.

G-I: Diarrhea

Cryptosporidium.	Protracted diarrhea, cholecystitis, cholangitis.	AFB stain of stool. Small bowel biopsy (stool may be ⊖).	Paromomycin. (octreotide).
Isospora.	Protracted diarrhea.	AFB stain of stool. Small bowel biopsy.	TMP-SMX.
Microsporidium.	Protracted diarrhea. (May also see cholecystitis, cholangitis, hepatitis, myositis).	Electron microscopy of small bowel Bx. Gram stain. Giemsa stain.	Metronidazole, albendazole.
Cyanobacteria-algae—Cyclospora.	Protracted diarrhea.	AFB stain of stool.	Possibly TMP-SMX.
MAC.	Diarrhea, fever, wt. loss malabsorption.	Biopsy. Stool culture *not* diagnostic of GI invasion.	Multi-drug regimen: Clarithromycin + ethambutol, ± rifampin ± ciprofloxacin. Primary prophylaxis (CD4 < 75): Rifabutin.
Salmonellosis.	Bacteremia, recurrence.	Blood and stool culture and sensitivity.	Ampicillin, TMP-SMX. Secondary prophylaxis: Cipro.
C. difficile.	Diarrhea, fever, abdominal pain.	Toxin assay, culture, endoscopy.	p.o. Vancomycin. (metronidazole)
CMV.	Diarrhea, ulcers, perforation.	Biopsy.	Ganciclovir. ?Benefit.
Shigella, Campylobacter.	Diarrhea, fever, abdominal pain.	Culture and sensitivity.	Ciprofloxacin.

(continued)

TABLE 13.4. (continued)

Syndrome	Etiology	Clinical	Diagnosis	Treatment
G-I: Diarrhea				
	Giardiasis.	Diarrhea.	Ova and parasite exam of stool or duodenal contents.	Metronidazole.
	Amebae.	Diarrhea, fever, abdominal pain.	Ova and parasite exam. Biopsy.	Metronidazole.
	HSV.	Diarrhea.	Biopsy.	Acyclovir.
	Strongyloidiasis.	Diarrhea, fever.	Ova and parasite exam of stool or duodenal contents.	Thiabendazole.
GI: Hepatobiliary				
Papillary stenosis. Sclerosing cholangitis.	Cryptosporidium. CMV. MAC.	Fever, pain, tenderness, ↑ alkaline phosphatase.	Sonogram. CT scan, ERCP.	Paromomycin. Ganciclovir. Clarithromycin + ethambutol ± rifampin ± ciprofloxacin.
Gangrenous cholecystitis.	CMV. Cryptosporidium. Candida.	Fever, pain.	Sonogram, HIDA scan.	Ganciclovir + surgery. Paromomycin + surgery. Amphotericin B + surgery.
Peliosis.	Bartonella.	Fever, pain.	Biopsy.	Erythromyin.

Neuro: Meningoencephalitis

Cryptococcus.	Meningoencephalitis; cryptococcoma.	CSF: CRAG, culture and sensitivity, India ink stain.	Amphotericin B ± 5-fluorocytosine (Fluconazole). Secondary prophylaxis: Fluconazole.
Toxoplasmosis.	Focal or diffuse findings; chorea helpful diagnostically.	Multiple lesions, ring-enhancing on CT or MRI (MRI most sensitive). PCR may prove useful.	Pyrimethamine and sulfadiazine (pyrimethamine and clindamycin). Primary prophylaxis (positive serology plus CD4 < 100/mm^3): TMP-SMX (dapsone and pyrimethamine). Secondary prophylaxis: pyrimethamine and sulfadiazine (also confers protection against PCP). (pyrimethamine and clindamycin).
TB.	Meningitis or tuberculoma or abscess ↑ protein, ↓ glucose.	TB elsewhere, CSF with lymphocytosis.	INH + rifampin + pyrazinamide + ethambutol. Steroids in severe disease. If MDR-TB suspected, use Amikacin + ofloxacin + ETH + PZA + possibly other drugs, pending culture results.

(continued)

TABLE 13.4. (continued)

Syndrome	Etiology	Clinical	Diagnosis	Treatment
Neuro: Meningoencephalitis				
	Progressive multifocal leukoencephalopathy (papovavirus-JC)	Focal deficits; limb weakness, visual loss, gait disturbance and headache, cognitive dysfunction.	MRI—scalloped hyperintense areas in white matter, without mass effect. Biopsy characteristic.	Experimental.
	HIV.	Aseptic meningitis. May be asymptomatic. Invades directly, during seroconversion phase or later. "AIDS Dementia"—cognitive, motor, then behavioral change.	Lymphs and ↑ protein in CSF.	Zidovudine (ZDV, AZT).
	Syphilis	Acute meningitis or meningovascular syphilis, e.g., CVA.	RPR, FTA-ABS, lymphs in CSF, protein ↑, serology may be falsely negative, glucose may be ↓.	Penicillin.
	Bacterial (Listeria, Meningococcus Pneumococcus, H. flu)	Fever, mental status change, headache, meningismus	Gram stain and culture of blood/CSF.	Per culture.

Neuro: cord-myelitis

	HIV, V-Z, HSV-2, toxo, CMV, TB, syphilis	Weakness, ataxia, hyperreflexia, incontinence, sensory loss, gait disturbance.	Lymphs, ↑ protein in CSF; on biopsy, white matter shows microvacuolation. R/O cord compression.	Per culture.
	HTLV-I-TSP	Spastic paraparesis, back pain.	Clinical; R/O cord compression.	None.

Neuro: cord-myelopathy

	Idiopathic.	Hyperreflexia, spasticity, incontinence.	CSF unremarkable, demyelination + vacuolization on biopsy, R/O cord compression.	None.

Neuro: Cranial Neuropathy

	Idiopathic.	C-VII. Usually resolves, may recur.	Clinical.	?

Neuro: Peripheral Neuropathy

	Inflammatory polyneuropathy, acute + chronic. Mononeuritis multiplex. Distal symmetric peripheral neuropathy.	↓DTRs, weakness, paresthesias.	Clinical. Exclude meds (ddI, ddC, INH).	?plasmapheresis.
	Autonomic neuropathy.	Orthostatic hypotension.	Clinical.	

(continued)

TABLE 13.4. *(continued)*

Syndrome	Etiology	Clinical	Diagnosis	Treatment
Skin				
Bacillary Angiomatosis.	Bartonella henselae. Bartonella quintana.	Papules, nodules, plaques; may clinically involve viscera.	Biopsy if necessary for silver stain, special culture, and PCR, if available.	Erythromycin.
Shingles.	V-Z virus.	Vesicles on red base. May include multiple contiguous dermatomes.	Clinical. Biopsy if necessary. Tzanck prep.	Acyclovir.
Molluscum contagiosum.	Virus.	Flesh colored papules with central umbilication.	Clinical.	Cantharidin, electrosurgery, cryosurgery.
Folliculitis.	Staphylococcus.	Pustules on face, trunk.	Clinical.	Dicloxacillin.
Cutaneous herpes.	HSV.	Group of vesicles which may → ulcers or necrosis.	Clinical; biopsy if necessary.	Acyclovir.
Mycobacterial infection.	MTB. MAC, *M. marinum* *M. hemophilum*, *M. kansasii*	Papules, pustules, plaques; may ulcerate.	Biopsy and culture and sensitivity.	Per culture & sensitivity.
Fungal Infection.	Histoplasmosis. Cryptococcosis. Coccidioidomycosis. Blastomycosis. Sporotrichosis. Paracoccidioidomycosis.	Combinations of pustules, plaques, nodules, ulcers; Crypto may resemble molluscum contagiosum.	Biopsy and culture.	Histo: amphotericin B. Secondary prophylaxis: itraconazole. Crypto: amphotericin B. Secondary prophylaxis: Fluconazole.

Scabies.	S. scabei.	Hyperkeratotic crusting.	Biopsy.	Cocci: amphotericin B. Secondary prophylaxis: Fluconazole. Blasto: itraconazole. Sporotrichosis: SSKI (itraconozole). Paracoccidioidomycosis: itraconazole. Kwell, Eurax.

Pulmonary

PCP.		Diffuse interstitial infiltrates; may cause abscess, effusion or focal abnormality.	Stain: BAL > induced sputum. Fluorescent antibody > Giemsa. Pulmonary function tests, Gallium scan, PCR if available.	Corticosteroids if PO_2 < 70 mm Hg. TMP-SMX (trimethoprim-dapsone or IV/IM pentamidine or atovaquone or clindamycin-primaquine). Primary prophylaxis (prior PCP, CD4 < 200/mm^3, thrush, FUO): TMP-SMX (dapsone or aerosolized pentamidine). Secondary prophylaxis: TMP-SMX (dapsone or aerosolized pentamidine).

(continued)

TABLE 13.4. (continued)

Syndrome	Etiology	Clinical	Diagnosis	Treatment
Pulmonary				
	TB.	"Routine" or hilar/mediastinal adenopathy, effusion, abscess. Atypical findings reflect ↓↓ CD_4 count.	Stain, culture and sensitivity of sputum.	INH + rifampin + ethambutol + pyrazinamide. If MDR-TB suspected treat pending culture results with Amikacin, ofloxacin, ETH and PZA, and possibly additional drugs. Prophylaxis: For PPD 5 mm, or contact: INH. For prophylaxis for MDR-TB: PZA + ofloxacin. For prophylaxis of INH-resistant organisms: RIF + ETH
	MAC.	Part of disseminated infection with wasting; interstitial infiltrates.	Stain, culture and sensitivity of sputum. Blood cultures.	Clarithromycin + ethambutol ± rifampin ± ciprofloxacin. Primary prophylaxis ($CD_4 < 75$): Rifabutin.
	Histoplasma.	Diffuse infiltrates. May cause hilar or mediastinal adenopathy.	Smear/culture and sensitivity of sputum. May see or grow from marrow or peripheral blood.	Amphotericin B. Secondary prophylaxis: itraconazole.
	Coccioides.	Diffuse infiltrates. May cause hilar or mediastinal adenopathy.	Culture or smear of sputum.	Amphotericin B. Secondary prophylaxis: Fluconazole.

	Cryptococcus.	Diffuse infiltrates or nodules; may cause adenopathy.	Sputum stain/culture and sensitivity, serum CRAG.	Ampho B, Fluconazole. Secondary prophylaxis: Fluconazole.
	Pneumococcus/H. Influenzae.	Like immunocompetent patients. Rarely diffuse infiltrates	Gm stain/culture and sensitivity of sputum. Blood cultures.	Third generation cephalosporin.
	CMV.	Diffuse interstitial infiltrates.	Biopsy. Culture of sputum or washings not sufficient for diagnosis.	Ganciclovir of ? benefit. May help to add immunoglobulin.
	Varicella-zoster.	Diffuse interstitial infiltrates. May be nodular.	Biopsy; culture and sensitivity.	Acyclovir.

Cardiac

Myocarditis.	Non-specific. Rare: viruses, cryptococcus, TOXO, TB.	CHF. Arrhythmias, chest pain.	Clinical.	Specific Rx for certain pathogens; corticosteroids.
Endocarditis.	Marantic.	Fever, petechiae, murmurs.	⊖ culture.	
	Staph in intravenous drug-abuser	Fever, petechiae, murmurs.	⊕ culture.	Vancomycin.
Effusion/tamponade.	MTB, MAC, cryptococcus.	↓ BP, ↓ Pulse pressure, signs of right heart failure	Echocardiogram. Pericardiocentesis + biopsy.	According to specific pathogen; drainage.

Myositis

(esp. psoas abscess).	Staphylococcus.	Pain, tenderness.	Biopsy, aspiration.	Antibiotic per culture/smear. Debridement.

(continued)

TABLE 13.4. (continued)

Syndrome	Etiology	Clinical	Diagnosis	Treatment
Sinusitis				
	H. Influenzae Pneumococcus Pseudomonas.	Fever, headache. (If < 200 CD_4 cells, multiple sinuses, often chronic, posterior sinus disease common.)	Aspiration.	Antibiotics per culture, decongestants.
Eye				
Retinitis.	Non-specific (50%).	Cotton-wool spots.	Clinical.	Resolves-no Rx necessary.
	CMV (25%). CD_4 < 50.	Hemmorhages and exudates.	Clinical.	Foscarnet. Ganciclovir (D/C AZT/ZDV) (need lifelong suppression).
	Toxo (rare).	Hemorrhages and exudates ass'd with vitritis and iritis (≠ CMV).	Clinical. Serology. PCR.	Pyrimethamine and sulfadiazine.
Endophthalmitis.	Candida and other fungi.	Pain, ↓vision.	Aspirate for Culture and sensitivity.	Ampho B.
Optic Neuritis.	Syphilis.	↓Vision. May have ass'd neurosyphilis.	Serology. Lumbar puncture.	Penicillin.
	Cryptococcosis.	Complicates cryptococcal meningitis.	Serology. Lumbar puncture. MRI.	Ampho B. ?Steroids. ?Decompression.

14

HEMATOLOGIC CHANGES ASSOCIATED WITH INFECTION

Some infections are characterized by changes in hematologic parameters. While never pathognomonic, such alterations may prove helpful in the differential diagnosis of infectious diseases.

CHANGES IN WBC

Increased WBC Count

Leukocytosis is an elevation in the wbc count. It is a non-specific finding and develops frequently in the course of many infectious and inflammatory disorders. There may be an associated neutrophilia (an increase in polymorphonuclear leukocytes, or PMNs), or a "shift to the left," an increase in the number of immature PMNs. All these leukocytic responses are non-specific and may be seen in most bacterial infections, some viral infections, and in many non-infectious disorders. However, a significant neutrophilia, with many bands, toxic granulations, vacuolization, and Döhle bodies, is an important clue to the presence of a severe bacterial infection. A shift to the left accompanied by a fall rather than a rise in WBC may be a particularly poor prognostic sign in many bacterial infections such as pneumococcal pneumonia.

Although leukocytosis is usually associated with neutrophilia, increased WBC counts may be seen with primarily a lymphocytosis. Pertussis, some cases of infectious mononucleosis caused by EBV (Epstein-Barr virus), CMV (cytomegalovirus), and toxoplasmosis may cause very high total WBC counts composed principally of lymphocytes.

Normal or Only Slightly Depressed WBC

Although leukocytosis is frequently a hallmark of infection, many infectious processes present with a normal or only slightly depressed WBC count. At times bacterial infections may show a "shift to the left" but no change in the total count. Neutrophilia without much total increase in the WBC also commonly occurs in leptospiral and rickettsial infections. In many viral infections and in a few bacterial infections such as typhoid fever and brucellosis, a normal or slightly low WBC accompanied by a relative lymphocytosis is observed. In malaria the count is usually normal, with a relatively normal differential.

Severely Depressed WBC

Acute infection with a severely depressed WBC count suggests the presence of one of these illnesses:

1. Overwhelming bacterial infection of any kind (e.g., seen in severe pneumococcal or Klebsiella pneumonia),
2. Overwhelming endotoxemia (e.g., Gram-negative bacteremia),
3. Miliary tuberculosis,
4. Certain viral infections, especially Colorado tick fever, lymphocytic choriomeningitis, or dengue,
5. Disseminated histoplasmosis,
6. Disseminated kala-azar.

Of course, a patient with a low total WBC count and infection may have another etiology for the leukocyte depression e.g., a primary hematologic process like leukemia, or leukopenia associated with drugs or toxins such as alcohol.

Lymphocytosis

Although a relative lymphocytosis may be present whenever PMLs are depressed, there is a group of conditions that may cause an absolute lymphocytosis:

1. Infectious mononucleosis (EBV infection)
2. CMV infection
3. Toxoplasmosis
4. Viral hepatitis
5. Many other viral infections
6. Pertussis
7. Brucellosis
8. Tuberculosis
9. Syphilis

All the illnesses listed above may also produce atypical lymphocytes, though the greatest atypical lymphocyte counts are seen with EB virus, CMV, and viral hepatitis. However, it should be remembered that atypical lymphocytes are also seen in some parasitic infections, especially toxoplasmosis and malaria, and are also common in the course of allergic reactions.

Monocytosis

Monocytosis may be seen as part of a chronic infectious process or during convalescence from an acute bacterial infection. Specific considerations include tuberculosis or other granulomatous infections, SBE (subacute bacterial endocarditis), or syphilis.

Eosinophilia

Eosinophilia is often an important clinical clue to the diagnosis of parasitic infestation. Trichinosis and visceral larva migrans are almost always associated with eosinophilia. On the other hand, in some parasitic infestations, including pinworm, whipworm, and amebiasis, eosinophilia is distinctly uncommon. When eosinophilia is present in one of these latter disorders, a search for other additional parasites should be made.

Eosinophilia may also occur as part of many chronic infections or may appear during convalescence from many bacterial diseases. Scarlet fever has been particularly associated with a late phase of eosinophilia. Deep fungal infections, especially coccidioidomycosis, sometimes produce eosinophilia. Numerous infectious disease processes and antimicrobial agents have been associated with eosinophilia and erythema nodosum. Eosinophilia associated with pulmonary infiltrates is associated with a variety of infectious (parasitic infection, tuberculosis, allergic aspergillosis) and noninfectious (asthma, vasculitis, sarcoid, lymphoma, drug allergy) disease states (See Chapter 2).

Eosinopenia

Acute, severe bacterial infections are almost always associated with eosinopenia. In fact, if the number of eosinophils in the peripheral smear is greater than 1 or 2 percent, one must be cautious in ascribing the illness to a bacterial infection. This clue must be interpreted with caution if the patient has other reasons for an elevated eosinophil count such as a coincident allergic reaction or parasitic infection.

CHANGES IN PLATELETS

Thrombocytopenia

Thrombocytopenia may occur with or without DIC (disseminated intravascular coagulation). Many kinds of serious infectious diseases have been associated with DIC. These include especially Gram-negative rod bacteremia, meningococcemia, and Rocky Mountain Spotted Fever. In patients with asplenia and pneumococcal bacteremia, DIC is frequent.

DIC is characterized by intravascular consumption of platelets and clotting factors. The consequences of this process are (a) a bleeding diathesis, (b) fibrinogen deposition in small vessels with resultant ischemic tissue damage, and (c) microangiopathic hemolytic anemia resulting from damage to the RBCs as they pass through the fibrin strands positioned across the lumina of small blood vessels.

Diagnosis of DIC is made or suspected by evaluation of the peripheral smear, platelet count, prothrombin time, partial thromboplastin time, fibrinogen level, measurement of fibrin degradation products, and assay of clotting factors V and VIII.

Thrombocytopenia without other evidence of DIC is especially common with RMSF and rubella, but may be seen with a wide variety of other infectious diseases.

Thrombocytosis

An increase in the absolute number of platelets is seen in many infectious processes, particularly in tuberculosis, in recovery from acute infection, and in some chronic infections, especially slowly resolving pneumonia.

CHANGES IN RBCs

Anemia is commonly seen in infectious disease states and is usually related to a combination of ineffective erythropoiesis and hemolysis. In many bacterial infections, mild hemolysis is present but not clinically apparent. However, hemolysis may be a serious component of the following infectious diseases:

1. *C. perfringens* toxemia, especially associated with septic abortion,
2. Malaria,
3. Babesiosis,
4. Bartonellosis,
5. Mycoplasmal pneumonia (rare cause) in convalescence,
6. Infectious mononucleosis (rare cause),
7. Syphilis.

In addition, marked hemolysis is sometimes seen in other viral diseases and with some bacteremias, especially those caused by staphylococci.

Infections may also cause hemolytic anemia by triggering an existing defect in the RBC. For example, a sickle cell hemolytic crisis may be set off by infection. Hemolysis may develop in a patient with G-6-PD deficiency because of an infection or the therapy administered. Sulfonamides, nitrofurantoin, chloramphenicol, primaquine, and aspirin are just a few of the drugs used in treating infectious diseases that are known to precipitate hemolysis in patients with G-6-PD deficiency.

Parvovirus B19 can cause transient RBC aplasia in patients with chronic hemolysis (e.g., sickle cell anemia). Rarely, parvovirus B19 produces RBC aplasia in normal patients. Immunodeficient patients infected with this virus, including those with AIDS, may develop profound RBC aplasia that responds to immunoglobulin therapy.

Pancytopenia results from infection causing a myelophthisic process, i.e., marrow replacement by diseases like tuberculosis or disseminated fungal infection. Also, pancytopenia may complicate hepatitis B and hepatitis C infections. The syndrome of hemophagocytosis, a proliferation of histocytes that phagocytize blood cells with resultant pancytopenia, has been attributed to a variety of infectious agents, including viruses (parvovirus B19, *Herpes simplex*, CMV, Varicella-zoster, EBV, adenovirus), *M. tuberculosis* (MTB), Leishmania, Babesia, and many bacteria and fungi.

SEDIMENTATION RATE

Although nonspecific, the sedimentation rate (ESR) is useful as an indication of acute infectious disease and as a means of following the progress of a patient under therapy. Acute illnesses without elevated ESRs are exceptions to the general rule. Thus on occasion, the observation of a normal or low ESR in an acutely ill patient may be extremely helpful. The ESR may be normal or low in an infectious process if severe hemolysis, DIC, or congestive heart failure is present. Certain infections such as trichinosis or viral hepatitis are especially notable for the lack of an elevation in the ESR.

15

SOURCES AND TRANSMISSION OF INFECTIOUS DISEASES OTHER THAN PERSON-TO-PERSON SPREAD

Many infectious diseases seen in the United States are transmitted to humans by means other than person-to-person spread. The following table (Table 15.1) lists the most important of these infections. This information may be used in two ways: one can check the various modes of acquiring a specific disease, or scan the infections that spread (a) by a specific mode of transmission, or (b) from a particular source.

For example, Brucellosis can be seen to spread by contact with animals, by ingestion of contaminated food, or via inhalation. Alternatively, the infections spread by ticks are easily identified as including arbovirus encephalitis, babesiosis, borreliosis, Colorado tick fever, ehrlichiosis, Lyme disease, Rocky Mountain spotted fever, and tularemia.

TABLE 15.1. SOURCES AND TRANSMISSION OF INFECTIOUS DISEASES OTHER THAN PERSON-TO-PERSON SPREAD

Disease	Direct Contact with Infected Animal or its Excreta	Ingestion of Contaminated Food or Water	Inhalation of Infected Dust or Aerosol	Mosquitoes	Flies	Ticks	Lice	Fleas	Mites
Amebiasis		X (human contamination)			X				
Anisakiasis		X							
Ascariasis		X							
Arbovirus encephalitis				X		X			
Babesiosis						X			
Borreliosis						X	X		
Brucellosis	X (pigs, cattle, sheep, goats, some dogs)	X (dairy products)	X						
Campylobacter	X	X							

TRANSMISSION OTHER THAN PERSON-TO-PERSON

Disease					
Cat-scratch disease	X (cat)				
Cholera		X (human contamination)			
Coccidioidomycosis			X		
Colorado tick fever					X
Cryptococcosis			X (pigeons)		
Cryptosporidium		X			
Dengue				X	
Diphyllobothrium		X			
E. coli		X			
Echinococcus		X			
Ehrlichiosis					X
Enterobiasis		X			

(continued)

DIFFERENTIAL DIAGNOSIS OF INFECTIOUS DISEASES

TABLE 15.1. *(continued)*

Disease	Direct Contact with Infected Animal or its Excreta	Ingestion of Contaminated Food or Water	Inhalation of Infected Dust or Aerosol	Mosquitoes	Flies	Ticks	Lice	Fleas	Mites
Giardiasis		X							
Hantavirus	X (mice)								
Hepatitis A & E		X (human contamination)							
Histoplasmosis			X (chicken, bat, starling)						
Legionellosis			X						
Leptospirosis	X (rats, pigs, cattle, others)	X (water)							
Listeria		X							
Lyme disease						X			
Lymphocytic choriomeningitis	X (mice hamsters)								

TRANSMISSION OTHER THAN PERSON-TO-PERSON

Disease	Col 1	Col 2	Col 3	Col 4	Col 5	Col 6
Malaria				X		
Melioidosis		X				
Murine typhus						X (rodents)
Plague			X			X (rodents)
Psittacosis			X (birds)			
Q fever	X (cattle, sheep)		X		Rare	
Rabies	X (dogs, cats, bats, foxes, skunks, others)				Rare	
Rat-bite fever (*Spirillum minus*)	X (rat)					
Rat-bite fever (*S. moniliformis*)	X (rat)	X				
Rickettsialpox						X (mouse)
Rocky Mountain spotted fever					X	

(continued)

TABLE 15.1. (continued)

Disease	Direct Contact with Infected Animal or its Excreta	Ingestion of Contaminated Food or Water	Inhalation of Infected Dust or Aerosol	Mosquitoes	Flies	Ticks	Lice	Fleas	Mites
Salmonellosis	X (poultry and numerous animals)	X (mammal or human contamination)			X				
Shigellosis	X (rare)	X (human contamination)			X				
Taenia solium and saginata		X							
Toxoplasmosis	X (cat)	X (meat)							
Trichinosis		X (meat)							
Tularemia	X (rabbits, muskrats)	X	X		X	X			
Typhus							X (human)	(flying squirrel)	
Yellow fever				X					

RECOMMENDED READING

CHAPTER 1. FEVER

Knockaert Daniel C, Vaneste Laurent J, Vaneste Stefand, Bobbaers Herman J. Fever of Unknown Origin in the 1980s. Arch Intern Med 1992; 152:51–56.

Saper Clifford B, Breder Christopher D. The Neurologic Basis of Fever. N Engl J Med 1994; 330:1880–86.

Simone Harvey B. Hyperthermia. N Engl J Med 1993; 329:83–88.

Styrt Barbara, Sugarman Barrett. Antipyresis and Fever. Arch of Intern Med 1990; 150:1589–97.

CHAPTER 2. PNEUMONITIS

Barnes Peter F, Barrows Susan A. Tuberculosis in the 1990s. Ann Intern Med 1993; 119:400–410.

Clyde Wallace A, Jr. Clinical Overview of Typical Mycoplasma Pneumoniae Infections. Clin Infect Dis 1993; 17 (Suppl 1):S32–6.

Marrie Thomas J. Community Acquired Pneumonia. Clin Infect Dis 1994; 18:501–15.

Martin Rebecca Edge, Bates Joseph H. Atypical Pneumonia. Infect Dis Clin N Am 1991; 585–602.

Nguyen M. Hung, Stout Janet E, Yu Victor L. Legionellosis. Infect Dis Clin of N Am. 1991; Sept 1:561–84.

Thom David H, Grayston J. Thomas. Infections with Chlamydia Pneumoniae Strain TWAR. Clinics Chest Med 1991; June 12:245–54.

CHAPTER 3. CEREBROSPINAL FLUID PLEOCYTOSIS

Halpern John J. Neuroborreliosis. Am J Med 1995; 98 (Suppl 4A): 52S-59S.

Harris Alan A, Levin Stuart. Brain Abscess. In: Gorbach Sherwood L, Bartlett John G, Blacklow Neil R. eds. Infectious Diseases. Philadelphia: WB Saunders, 1992.

Kasik John E. Central Nervous System Tuberculosis. In Schlossberg David ed. Tuberculosis. 3rd ed. New York: Springer-Verlag, 1994; 129-142.

Quagliarello Vincent J, Scheld W Michael. New Perspectives on Bacterial Meningitis. Clin Infect Dis 1993; 17:603-10.

Swartz Morton N. Neurosyphilis. In: Holmes Kin K, Mardh Per-Anders, Sparling P Frederick, Wiesner Paul J, Cates Willard Jr, Lemon Stanley M, Stamm Walter E, eds. Sexually Transmitted Diseases. 2nd ed. New York: McGraw-Hill, 1990; 231-246.

CHAPTER 4. BACTERURIA AND PYURIA

Chanel George G, Harding Godfrey KM, Guay David R.P. Asymptomatic Bacteruria. Arch Intern Med 1990; 150:1389-1396.

Kunin Calvin M. Urinary Tract Infections in Females. Clin Infect Dis 1994; 18:1-12.

McCormack Rein Michael F. Urethritis. In: Mandell Gerald L, Bennett John E, Dolin Raphael. Principles and Practice of Infectious Diseases, Fourth Edition. New York: Churchill-Livingstone, 1995.

Pezzlo Marie T. Laboratory Diagnosis of Urinary Tract Infection: current concepts and controversies. Infect Dis Clin Pract 1994; 2:469-472.

Stamm Walter E, Hooton Thomas M. Management of Urinary Tract Infections in Adults. N Engl J Med 1993; 329:1328-1334.

Storfer Stephen P, Medoff Gerald, Fraser Victoria J, Powderly William G, Dunagan William Clayborne. Candiduria: Retrospective Review in Hospitalized Patients. Infect Dis Clin Pract 1994; 3:23-29.

CHAPTER 5. DIARRHEA

Adal Karim A. From Wisconsin to Nepal: cryptosporidium, cyclospora and microsporidia. Curr Opin Infect Dis 1994; 7:609-615.

Bartlett John G. Antibiotic Associated Diarrhea. Clin Infect Dis 1992; 15: 573-81.

Blacklow Neil R, Greenberg Harry B. Viral Gastroenteritis. N Engl J Med 1991; 325:252-264.

DuPont Herbert L, Ericsson Charles D. Prevention and Treatment of Traveler's Diarrhea. N Engl J Med 1993; 328: 1821–1828.

Guerrant Richard L, Bobak David A. Bacterial and Protozoal Gastroenteritis. N Engl J Med 1991; 325:327–340.

Hill Michael K, Sanders Charles V. Localized and Systemic Infection due to Vibrio Species. Infect Dis Clin N Amer 1987; 1:687–707.

Theilmen Nathan M. Enteric Escherichia Coli Infections. Curr Opin Infect Dis 1994; 7:582–591.

CHAPTER 6. RASH

Cherry James D. Contemporary Infectious Exanthems. Clin Infect Dis 1993; 16:199–207.

Farrar W Edmond, Wood Martin J, Innes John A, Tubbs Hugh. Infectious Diseases Text and Color Atlas. 2nd ed. New York: Gower Medical Publishing, 1992.

Fitzpatrick Thomas B, Johnson Richard Allen, Polanomachiel K, Suurmond Dick, Wolff Klaus. Color Atlas and Synopsis of Clinical Dermatology. 2nd ed. New York: McGraw-Hill, 1992.

Myers Sarah A, Sexton Daniel J. Dermatologic Manifestations of Arthropod Borne Diseases. Infect Dis Clin of N Amer 1994; 8:689–712.

Stevens Dennis L. Invasive Group A Streptococcus Infections. Clin Infect Dis 1992; 14:2–13.

Stevens Dennis L, Bryant Amy E, Hackett Shawn P. Sepsis Syndromes and Toxic Shock Syndromes: concepts and pathogenesis and a perspective of future treatment strategies. Curr Opin Infect Dis 1993; 6: 374–383.

CHAPTER 7. MONOARTHRITIS

Baker Daniel G, Schumacher H Ralph Jr. Acute Monoarthritis. N Engl J Med 1993; 329:1013–1020.

McCarty Daniel J, Koopman William J. Arthritis and Allied Conditions. Philadelphia: Lea and Febiger, 1993.

CHAPTER 8. POLYARTHRITIS

Fink Chester W. Reactive Arthritis. Ped Infect Dis J 1988; 7:58–65.

Pinals Robert S. Polyarthritis and Fever. N Engl J Med 1994; 330: 769–774.

Stere Alan C, Schoen Robert T, Taylor Elias E. The Clinical Evolution of Lyme Arthritis. Ann Intern Med 1987; 107:725–731.

Woplf Anthony D, Campion Jiles V, Chishick Alice, et al. Clinical Manifestations of Human Parvovirus B19 in Adults. Arch Intern Med 1989; 149:1153–1156.

CHAPTER 9. JAUNDICE

Marton Keith I, Doubliet Peter. How to Image the Gallbladder in Suspected Cholecystitis. Ann Intern Med 1988; Nov. 722–730.

Sherlock Sheila, Dooley James. Jaundice. In: Diseases of the Liver and Biliary System. 9th Edition. Blackwell Scien Publ Oxford, 1993: 199–214.

Shu Henry H, Feinstone Steven M, Hoofnagle JH. Hepatitis. In: Mandell Gerald L, Bennett John E, Dolan Raphael, eds. Principles and Practice of Infectious Diseases. New York: Churchill-Livingstone, 1995; 136–1153.

Sinanan Mika N. Acute Cholangitis. Infect Dis Clin N Amer 1992; 6: 571–600.

Hau Toni. Infections of the Liver and Spleen. In: Howard Richard J, Simmons Richard L, eds. Surgical Infectious Disease. 3rd ed. Connecticut: Appleton & Lange, 1995; 1031–1058.

CHAPTER 10. SPLENOMEGALY

Erslev Allan J. Hypersplenism and Hyposplenism. In: Williams William J, Beutler Ernest, Erslev Allan J, Lichtman Marshall A, eds. Hematology. 4th Ed. New York: McGraw-Hill, 1990.

Neva Franklina A, Brown Harold W. Basic Clinical Parasitology 6th Ed. Norwalk, Connecticut: Appleton and Lange, 1994:81–103 (Malaria).

Strouse Stephen E, Cohen Jeffrey I, Tosato Giovanna, Mier Jeffrey. Epstein Barr Infections: Biology, Pathogenesis, and Management. Ann Intern Med 1993; 118:45–58.

Hart F Dudley ed. French's Index of Differential Diagnosis 12th ed. Chicago: Yearbook Medical Publishing, 1985.

CHAPTER 11. LYMPHADENOPATHY

Adal Karim A, Cockerill Clay J, Petri William A Jr. Cat Scratch Disease, bacillary angiomatosis and other infections due to Rochalimaea. N Engl J Med 1994; 330:1509–1516.

Brook Itzhak. Pharyngotonsillitis. In: Cunha Burke A, ed. Infectious Disease Practice. New York: MBC Publications Inc., 1994.

Dylewski Joseph, Berry Gerald, Pham-Dang Huong. Unusual Cause of Cervical Lymphadenitis: Kikuchi-Fujimoto Disease. Rev Infect Dis 1991; 13:823–5.

Freidig EE, McClure SP, Wilson WR, Banks PM, Washington II, JA. Clinical-Histologic-Microbiologic Analysis of 419 Lymph Node Biopsy Specimens. Rev Infect Dis. 1986; 8:322–328.

Margileth Andrew M, Hayden Gregory F. Cat Scratch Disease (Editorial). N Engl J Med 1993; 329:53–54.

Piot Peter, Plummer Francis A. Genital Ulcer Adenopathy Syndrome. In: Holmes King K, Mardh Per-Andes, Sparling P Frederick, Wiesner Paul J, Cates Willard Jr, Lemon Stanley M, Stamm Walter E, eds. Sexually Transmitted Diseases. 2nd ed. New York: McGraw-Hill, 1990; 711–716.

CHAPTER 12. INFECTION IN THE COMPROMISED HOST

Claman Henry N. The Biology of the Immune Response. J Amer Med Assoc 1992; 268:2790–2796.

Karp Judith E, Merz William G, Dick James D. Management of Infections in Neutropenic Patients: advances in therapy and prevention. Curr Opin Infect Dis 1993; 6:405–411.

Pizzo Philip A. Management of Fever in Patients with Cancer and Treatment Induced Neutropenia. N Engl J Med 1993; 328:1323–1332.

Sable Carole A, Donowitz Gerald R. Infections in Bone Marrow Transplant Recipients. Clin Infect Dis 1994; 18:273–84.

Walzer Peter D, Wimbey Estella. Overview of Prevention of Infections in The Immunocompromised Patient. Clin Infect Dis 1993; 17 (Suppl 2): S376–7.

CHAPTER 13. AIDS

Bartlett John G. Prevention of Opportunistic Infections in Human Immunodeficiency Virus Infected Patients. Infect Dis Clin Pract 1994; 3: 260–269.

Glaser Carolanne, Angulo Frederick James, Rooney J Aline. Animal Associated Opportunistic Infections Among Persons Infected with the Immunodeficiency Virus. Clin Infect Dis 1994; 18:14–24.

Sande Merle A, Volberding Paul A. The Medical Management of AIDS. 4th ed. Philadelphia: WB Saunders Co, 1995.

Moe Ardis A, Hardy W David. Pneumocystis Carinii Infection in HIV-Sero-positive Patients. Infect Dis Clin N Amer 1994; 8:331–364.

Revised Classification System for HIV Infection and Expanded Surveillance Case Definition for AIDS. MMWR Dec. 18, 1992; 41:No RR–14.

CHAPTER 14. HEMATOLOGIC CHANGES

Anderson Larry J. Human Parvoviruses. J Infect Dis 1990; 161:603–608.

Marder Victor J. Consumptive Thrombohemorrhagic Disorders. In: Williams William J, Beutler Ernest, Erslev Allen J, Lichtman Marshall A. eds. Hematology. 4th ed. New York: McGraw-Hill, 1990; 1522–1542.

Rinier Alexander P, Spivak Gerry L. Hematophagocytic Histiocystosis. A report of 23 new patients and a review of the literature. Medicine 1988; 67:369–388.

INDEX

Abscess (es)
　brain
　　not ruptured, 78–79t
　　ruptured, 62, 65, 76–77t
　cerebral epidural, 66, 78–79t
　hepatic, 201–202
　　amebic, 202, 211t
　　pyogenic, 201–202, 209–210t
　outside the GU tract, 98
　perinephric, 97, 110t
　posterior epidural, 67
　renal, 96–97, 109t
　search for, 6–7, 9t
　spinal epidural, 67, 78–79t
　splenic, 218
Acanthameba, 62
Achronosis, 180t
Acid fast stains, 122
Acquired Immunodeficiency Syndrome. See AIDS
Actinomycosis, and pneumonia, 14t
Acute endocarditis (ABE), and splenomegaly, 214
Acyclovir, 70, 71
　for pneumonia, 28t, 49t

Adenovirus, 117
　and viral pneumonia, 24, 25
AIDS
　antiretroviral therapy, 283
　associated organisms, 268t
　cardiac syndromes, 287, 299t
　classification systems for HIV infection, 281, 281t
　constitutional syndromes, 283, 285–287
　　cryptococcus, 283, 289t
　　histoplasma, 283, 288t
　　Kaposi's sarcoma, 285, 289t
　　M. Avium complex (MAC), 283, 288t, 298t
　　M. tuberculosis (MTB), 283, 288t
　　non-Hodgkin's lymphoma, 285, 289t
　course of HIV infection and CD4 cell count, 280
　CSF pleocytosis, 286
　dementia complex, 285
　dermatologic manifestations, 286, 296–297t

320 INDEX

AIDS—continued
  diagnosis and management, 281, 283
  and EB virus, distinguishing, 280
  gastrointestinal syndromes
    cytomegalovirus (CMV), 285, 289t
    diarrhea, 122, 285, 291–292t
    hairy leukoplakia, 285, 289t
    hepatobiliary syndromes, 285, 292t
    herpes simplex virus (HSV), 285, 289t
    histoplasma, 285, 289t
  incubation period, 279
  infectious complications by syndromes, 283, 284t, 288–300t
  meningitis and, 64
  myositis, 299t
  neurologic syndromes
    cord-myelitis, 286, 295t
    cord-myelopathy, 286, 295t
    cranial neuropathy, 286, 295t
    meningoencephalitis, 285–286, 293–294t
    peripheral neuropathy, 286, 295t
  ophthalmologic complications, 287, 300t
  pseudoappendicitis in, 285
  pulmonary syndromes, 286–287, 298–299t
  pneumonia, 26, 48t, 286
  recommended reading, 317–318
  at risk populations, 279
  side effects of therapy, 282–283
  sinusitis, 287, 300t
  Surveillance Case definition, 281, 282t
Allergic reaction, and rashes, 148, 149t
Alveolar proteinosis, associated organisms, 267t
Amantidine, for pneumonia, 28t

Amebiasis, 146t
  and diarrhea, 122–123, 132t
  transmission of, 308t
Amebic meningitis, 62, 76–77t
Amikacin, for pneumonia, 31t, 34t
Aminoglycoside, for pneumonia, 30t
Amphotericin B, 62, 101
  for pneumonia, 41t, 42t, 43t, 46t, 47t, 48t
Ampicillin, 60, 148
  for management of UTI, 99
  for pneumonia, 31t
Amyloidosis, 180t, 218t
Anaerobic pneumonia, 19–20, 23, 31–33t
Anaphylatoxin, 263
Anemia, 305
Angiography, 7
Angiomatosis, and AIDS, 296t
Animal populations, encephalitis in, 72
Anisakiasis, transmission of, 308t
Anopheles mosquito, 217
Anthrax, 146t
Antibiotic therapy
  for FUO, 7, 8
  for prostatitis, 100
Antibiotic-induced diarrhea, 123–124
Anticoagulants, 67
Anticoagulation therapy, pulmonary embolism, 50t
Anti-infective agents, causing jaundice, 195, 197
Antimicrobial therapy
  in the compromised host, 270
  for management of UTI, 99
Antinuclear antibody studies, 6, 10t
Antiretroviral therapy, AIDS, 283
Antituberculosis therapy, 7
Aortic regurgitation, 174
Appendicitis, 120, 201
Arachidonic acid, 1
Arbovirus (es), 71, 72
Arbovirus arthritis, 177

INDEX

Arbovirus encephalitis,
  transmission of, 308t
Arcanobacterium hemolyticum, 147,
  230, 243t
Arteritis, cerebral, 63
Arthralgias, 171
Arthritis. *See* Monoarthritis;
  Polyarthritis
Ascariasis, transmission of, 308t
"Aseptic" meningitis, 64, 73, 73t
Aspergillus, and pneumonia in the
  compromised host, 15t, 26,
  46t
Aspiration, 25
Asymptomatic bacteriuria, 98–99
Atrial myxoma, 174
Augmentin, for management of
  UTI, 99
Azathioprine, and CSF pleocytosis,
  73t
AZT, 283

B. burgdorferi, 178
B. cereus, and diarrhea, 118, 128t
Babesiosis
  and jaundice, 197
  transmission of, 308t
Bacteremia, 201
  and AIDS, 289t
  and jaundice, 201
  rash, 139, 152–153t
  and splenomegaly, 214
Bacteria, associated with humoral
  or T-cell defects, 266t
Bacterial adenitis, 232–233, 246t
Bacterial arthritis, 168t
Bacterial endocarditis
  CSF count, 67, 82–83t
  and "Osler's triad," 67
  and polyarthritis, 174, 183–184t
  rash, 137, 150–151t
Bacterial meningitis, 74–75t
  age-related pathogens, 57
  diagnostic studies to detect
    etiology of, 60, 61t
  H. influenzae meningitis, 59

meningococcal and
  meningococcemia, 58
other causes of, 59–60
partially treated, 65, 76–77t
pneumococcal, 57–58
Bacterial pneumonia, 14t, 16
Bacteriuria. *See* Urinary tract
  infection (UTI)
Bacteroides fragilis, 201
Bactrim, 60, 99
Baker's cysts, 178
Balanitis, 90
Bartonella henselae, 233
Bartonellosis, 198
Behcet's syndrome, 180t
  and CSF pleocytosis, 84–85t73t
Bell's Palsy, 72
Berylliosis, 218t
Beta-hemolytic streptococci, and
  septic arthritis in children,
  163
Biopsy
  lung, 27
  open-lung, 8
  sites, 6
Bladder irrigation, 101
Blastomyces dermatitidis, cause of
  monoarthritis, 166
Blastomycosis, 64, 146t, 234
  and pneumonia, 14t
Bleomycin therapy, causing FUO, 8
Blood cultures, for pneumonia
  diagnosis, 22
Borelliosis, transmission of, 308t
Botulism, 124
Bradycardia, and pneumonia, 26
Branhamella catarrhalis, 19
Brill-Zinsser disease, rash, 140, 142
Bronchoscopy, for pneumonia
  diagnosis, 23
Brucellosis, 5, 237, 258t
  and pneumonia, 14t, 26
  transmission of, 308t
Bruton's hypogammaglobulinemia,
  262
Bubonic plague, 234
Burns, associated organisms, 267t

C. albicans, and cystitis, 95
C. difficile, -related diarrhea, 120, 123, 131t
C. perfringens, 116t, 117, 127t
 and jaundice, 197–198, 203t
Campylobacter
 and Reiter's syndrome, 173
 transmission of, 308t
Campylobacter jejuni infection, and diarrhea, 120, 131t
Candida
 and AIDS, 289t, 290t
 and pneumonia in the compromised host, 15t, 26, 46t
Candidal urethritis, 92, 103t
Carbamazepine, and CSF pleocytosis, 73t
Cardiac syndromes, in AIDS, 287, 299t
CAT scan, 6, 9t
Catheters, indwelling IV, infections from, 139
Cat-scratch disease, 233, 246–247t
 transmission of, 309t
CD8 lymphocytes, 176
CD4 T-cell count, 280–281
CDC staging system, for HIV infection, 281
Cefotaxime, 58
 for pneumonia, 29t
Ceftriaxone, for pneumonia, 38t
Cellulitis, 233
 etiology, 145t
Cephalosporin, for pneumonia, 29t, 30t
Cerebral infarction, 2
Cerebrospinal fluid pleocytosis
 acid-fast smears of CSF, increasing yield on, 63
 basics types of, 54, 56, 56t
 diagnosis of CNS infection, 53
 evaluation of CNS infection, 54
 noninfectious causes of, 73, 73t, 84–85t
 nontreatable infections, type C CSF findings, 71–73, 82–83t
 recommended reading, 314
 symptoms and signs of CNS infection, 53
 treatable infections
  type A CSF findings, 56–63, 74–75t
   amebic meningitis, 62, 76–77t
   bacterial meningitis
    age-related pathogens, 57
    diagnostic studies to detect etiology of, 60, 61t
    H. influenzae meningitis, 59
    meningococcal and meningococcemia, 58
    other causes of, 59–60
    pneumococcal, 57–58
    ruptured brain abscess, 62, 76–77t
  type B CSF findings
   fungal meningitis, 64, 76–77t
   tuberculosis meningitis, 62–63, 76–77t
  type C CSF findings
   "aseptic" meningitis, 64
   herpes simplex types 1&2, meningoencephalitis, 70–71, 82–83t
   Leptospiral meningitis, 69, 80–81t
   Lyme disease, 68–69, 80–81t
   malaria, 69–70, 80–81t
   parameningeal infections, 65–68, 78–79t
   partially treated bacterial meningitis, 65, 76–77t
   syphilitic meningitis, 68–69, 78–79t
   toxoplasmosis, 70, 80–81t
   trichinosis, 70, 80–81t
Cervical adenitis, 229–232
Cervicitis, 90
Chancroid, 235, 251t

Charcot's biliary fever, 5, 198
Charcot's joints, 178
Chemotaxis, 263
Chemotherapy, and FUO, 8
Chikungunya fever, 177
Chlamydia, and Reiter's syndrome, 173
Chlamydia pneumoniae, 14t, 16, 21, 35t
Chlamydia trachomatis, 14t, 15, 90, 92
Chloramphenicol, 140
 for pneumonia, 37t
Chloroquine, for pneumonia, 45t
Cholangitis, 198
 and jaundice, 205t
Cholecystitis, 198–199
 and jaundice, 198–199, 204t
Cholecystostomy, 199
Cholelithiasis, chronic, 199
Cholera
 and diarrhea, 117, 127t
 transmission of, 309t
CIE, 60, 61t
Ciprofloxacin, and CSF pleocytosis, 73t
Cirrhosis, 218t
 associated organisms, 267t
Clindamycin, 31t, 283 Clostridial diarrhea, 117
Clostridium septicum, 20
Clutton's joints, 178
CMV. *See* Cytomegalovirus (CMV)
Coccidioides immitis, 64, 166
Coccidioidomycosis, 64, 234
 and pneumonia, 14t
 and polyarthritis, 176–177, 187t
 transmission of, 309t
Collagen vascular disease, 5, 175
 search for, 5, 10t
Colorado tick fever. *See* Rocky Mountain spotted fever (RMSF)
Complement cascade deficiencies, 262–263

Compromised host
 abnormalities of PML function, 263, 264–265t
 candidiasis, 265, 272–273t
 CMV infection, 277t
 cryptococcosis, 273t
 defects in host defense
  defects of the cell-mediated immune system, 263
  impaired humoral immunity, or phagocytosis, 262–263
  mechanical barriers, 261–262
  suppressed normal flora, 262
 diagnosis, establishing, 269
 general therapeutic guidelines, 269–270
 herpes simplex infection, 278t
 invasive aspergillosis, 273t
 listeriosis, 275t
 mycotic infection, 265, 272t
 nocardiosis, 274–275t
 opportunistic pathogens, 265–266
  associated with humoral or T-cell defects, 266t
  associated with particular medical conditions, 267–268t
 P. carinii, 275t
 phycomycosis, 274t
 pneumonia in, 26–27, 46–48t
 preventive measures, 270–271
 pulmonary infiltrate, 268
 recommended reading, 317
 strongyloides hyperinfection syndrome, 276t
 toxoplasmosis, 276t
 varicella-zoster infection, 276–277t
 vaccination and, 271
Congestive heart failure, 218t
Cord-myelitis, and AIDS, 286, 295t
Cord-myelopathy, and AIDS, 286, 295t
Coronary arteritis, 147
Coxsackie virus, 72

Cranial nerve palsies, 69
Cranial neuropathy, and AIDS, 286, 295t
Crohn's disease, 120
Cryptococcus
　and AIDS, 283, 289t, 299t
　and pneumonia in the compromised host, 15t, 27, 47t
　transmission of, 309t
Cryptococcus neoformans, 64
Cryptosporidium, 122, 128t
　transmission of, 309t
Culture-negative endocarditis, 174
Cutaneous herpes, and AIDS, 296t
Cyanobacteria, 122
Cyclospora, 122, 128t
Cyst (s), 218t
Cystic duct obstruction, 199
Cystic fibrosis, associated organisms, 267t
Cystitis, 94–95, 106–107t, 110–111t
Cystoscopy, 95
Cytolysis, 263
Cytomegalovirus (CMV), 5, 123, 200, 216, 236, 254t
　and AIDS, 280, 290t, 299t
　and pneumonia, in the compromised host, 14t
　and viral pneumonia, 25

Dementia complex, AIDS, 285
Dengue, 3, 236–237, 255t
　transmission of, 309t
Dermatologic manifestations, AIDS, 286, 296–297t
Diabetes mellitus, 218t
Diabetic ketoacidosis, associated organisms, 267t
Diarrhea
　and AIDS, 292t
　causes of diarrheal diseases
　　antibiotic-induced diarrhea, 123–124
　　inflammatory
　　　Campylobacter jejuni
　　　infection, 120, 131t
　　invasive infections: enteroinvasive *E. coli* (EIEC), 119
　　invasive infections: Shigellosis, 118–119, 129t
　　penetrating (enteric fever), 121
　　salmonellosis, 119, 129t
　　staphylococcal enterocolitis, 120
　　Vibrio parahaemolyticus, 120–121
　　Yersinia enterocolitica infection, 119, 129t
　noninfectious causes of diarrhea, 125t
　noninflammatory, 116t
　　B. cereus, 118, 128t
　　cholera, 117
　　clostridial diarrhea, 117
　　enterotoxigenic *E. coli* (ETEC), 117–118, 126–127t
　　staphylococcal food poisoning, 117
　　viral gastroenteritis, 116–117, 126t
　parasitic, 121–122
　　amebiasis, 122–123, 132t
　　giardiasis, 123, 128t
　toxin-induced gastroenteritis, 124, 125t
　defined, 113
　general features
　　fecal leukocytes, 115
　　host factors, 115
　　inflammatory diarrhea, 113–114, 114t
　　noninflammatory diarrhea, 113, 114t
　　penetrating diarrhea, 114t, 114–115
　non-specific therapy for, 124
　recommended reading, 314–315
　traveler's, 122
Didanosine (ddI), 283

Diphtheria, 146t
  and acute cervical lymphadenopathy, 231, 242t
Diphyllobothrium, transmission of, 309t
Diseases, systemic, that cause fever, 5
Disseminated intravascular coagulation (DIC), 136–137, 156–157t, 304–305
Diverticulitis, 201
DNA probes, for pneumonia diagnosis, 23
Double quotidian fever, 3
Doxycycline, 35t, 36t
  for pneumonia, 38t, 39t
Drug fever, 7–8
Drug reactions, causing rash, 147–148
Drugs
  CSF findings, 73, 73t, 84–85t
  hypersensitivity to, 218t
  side effects of, in AIDS patients, 281, 283
  that produce jaundice, 197

E. coli, 201
  and cystitis, 94
  and diarrhea, 113, 114t
  and pneumonia, 18
  and prostatitis, 93
  transmission of, 309t
E. histolytica
  and diarrhea, 122–123
  and pneumonia, 14t
EB virus. See Epstein-Barr virus (EBV)
Echinococcus, 219
  transmission of, 309t
ECHO type 9, rash, 140
Echovirus, 72
Ecthyma, 146t
"Ecthyma gangrenosum," 139
Effusion/tamponade, and AIDS, 299t

Ehrlichiosis
  rash, 142, 147
  transmission of, 309t
Elderly, febrile response to infection, 2
ELISA, 60, 61t
Empyema, subdural, 66
Encephalopathy, toxic, 67–68, 82–83t
Endocarditis, 3, 5
  and AIDS, 299t
  search for, 9t
  See also Bacterial endocarditis
Endocrinopathies, associated organisms, 267t
Endophthalmitis, and AIDS, 300t
Enteric fever, 121
Enteric infections, 114t
Enterobacter
  and cystitis, 94
  and meningitis, 59
Enterobiasis, transmission of, 309t
Enterococci
  and cystitis, 94
  and prostatitis, 93
Enterohemorrhagic E. coli (EHEC), 118
Enteroinvasive E. coli (EIEC), and diarrhea, 119
Enterotoxigenic E. coli (ETEC), and diarrhea, 117–118, 126–127t
Enterotoxin B or C, 145
Enterovirus, 71, 72, 117
Eosinopenia, 304
Eosinophilia, 202, 303–304
Epidermolysins A and B, 145, 147
Epididymitis, and prostatitis, 93
Epstein-Barr virus (EBV), 5, 71, 72, 200, 230
  and AIDS, 290t
  and splenomegaly, 216, 222t
Erythema (s), rash, 144–145, 147, 158–159t
Erythema chronicum migrans, 69, 143, 178
Erythema infectiosum, 175–176

326 INDEX

Erythema nodosum, 119, 177
Erythromycin, for pneumonia, 28t, 35t, 39t, 40t
Esophagitis, and AIDS, 290–291t
Ethambutol, 7

Factious fever, 3–4
Familial Mediterranean fever, 180t
Fecal leukocytes, 115, 117
Felty's syndrome, 218t
Fever
  body temperature, normal variations in, 1–2
  classification of, 3
  common pathways in production of, 1
  drug fever, 7–8
  factitious fever, 3–4
  fever of undetermined origin (FUO), 3
    infectious causes of, 5–6
    laboratory procedures, studies and workups, for evaluating, 6–7, 9–11t
    noninfectious causes of, 6
    therapeutic trials, 7
  in hospitalized patients, 7–8
  in the immunosuppressed patient, 8
  in non-hospitalized patients, 3–7
  noninfectious causes of, 3
  pathological causes of, 2
  patient with, 4t
  patterns of, 2–3
  physiologic states that cause, 2
  psychogenic, 7
  recommended reading, 313
  site specific pathogens, antibiotic therapy against, 88
  specific disease patterns, 3
Fifth disease, 175–176
Fish poisoning, and diarrhea, 124
Fitzhugh-Curtis syndrome, 199, 205–206t
Fluconazole, 101, 283
5-flurocytosine, for pneumonia, 46t, 47t

Folliculitis, and AIDS, 296t
Fungi/fungal infections
  and AIDS, 296t
  associated with humoral or T-cell defects, 266t
  fungal meningitis, 64, 76–77t
  fungal pyelonephritis, 96
  and monoarthritis, 166, 168t
  and pneumonia, 14t, 26, 40–43t
  and pneumonia, in the compromised host, 15t
Fungus balls, and UTI, 101
Fusospirochetal infection, and pharyngitis, 231, 243t

Gamma globulin, and CSF pleocytosis, 73t
Ganciclovir, for pneumonia, 28t, 49t
Gangrene, acral, 140
Gentamicin
  for management of UTI, 99
  for pneumonia, 31t
Giardia lamblia, 123
Giardiasis
  and diarrhea, 122, 123, 128t
  transmission of, 310t
"Gibbus," 165
Gomori silver stain, 229
Gonococcal arthritis, 171–173, 181t
Gonococcal endocarditis, 3
Gonococcal monoarthritis, 164, 164t
Gonococcal perihepatitis, and jaundice, 199, 205–206t
Gonococcal pharyngitis, 230, 243t
Gonococcal urethritis, 92, 102t
Gonococcemia, rash, 138, 144, 152–153t
Gout, 166, 167t, 168t, 180t
G-6-PD deficiency, 198, 306
Gram stain, for pneumonia diagnosis, 22–23
Gram-negative bacilli pneumonia, 18, 30t

INDEX

Gram-negative rods
  aerobic, 202
  and septic arthritis in children, 163, 165
Gram-positive cocci, 202
  and monoarthritis, 164
Granulatomous disease, associated organisms, 267t
Granulocytopenia, 270
Granuloma inguinale, 236, 252t
Grave's disease, 218t
Group A streptococcal pharyngitis, 229, 240–241t
Gummatous joints, 178

H. capsulatum, 219
H. influenzae, 15
  and AIDS, 299t
  meningitis, 59
  and septic arthritis in children, 163
Haemophilus pneumonia, 20, 29t
Hantavirus, transmission of, 310t
Harmartomas, 218t
Haverhill fever, 178
Heat stroke, 2
Heavy metals, and diarrhea, 124
Helicobacter pylori, 123
Helminths, 122
Hemarthrosis, causing monoarthritis, 167t
Hematologic changes associated with infection
  eosinopenia, 304
  eosinophilia, 303–304
  lymphocytosis, 303
  monocytosis, 303
  platelets, changes in
    thrombocytopenia, 304–305
    thrombocytosis, 305
  RBCs, changes in, 305–306
  recommended reading, 318
  sedimentation rate, 306
  WBC count
    increased, 301–302

    normal or slightly depressed, 302
    severely depressed, 302
Hematuria, 174
Hemoglobinopathy, 180t, 218t
Hemolysis, 305–306
Hemolytic anemia, 218t
Hemolytic states, associated organisms, 267t
Hemophagocytosis, 306
Hemorrhage, subarachnoid, and CSF pleocytosis, 73t
Hepatitis, 5, 237
  alcoholic, 199
  infectious, 199
  and jaundice, 200–202
  transmission of, 310t
Hepatobiliary syndromes, AIDS, 292–293t
Herpangina, 72
Herpes hominis, and pneumonia in the compromised host, 14t
Herpes simplex virus (HSV), 92, 146t, 200, 236, 252t
  and AIDS, 289t, 290t
  and meningoencephalitis, 70–71, 82–83t
  rash, 144
Herpes virus, and viral pneumonia, 24, 25
Herpes zoster
  infection, 234, 249t
  rash, 144
Herpetic whitlow, 234, 235, 250t
HHV-6, 237
Histiocytosis, 218t
Histoplasma, and AIDS, 283, 288t, 298t
Histoplasmosis, 64, 237–238, 259t
  and pneumonia, 14t
  and splenomegaly, 219, 220–221t
  transmission of, 310t
HIV infection, 200, 237, 259t
  and polyarthritis, 176, 186t
  See also AIDS
HLA-B27 positivity, 176

Hodgkin's disease, 3, 8
and pneumonia, 26
Horder's spots, 143, 217
Human immunodeficiency virus.
See AIDS; HIV
Hydrarthrosis, 178
Hyperbilirubinemia, and jaundice, 195
Hypergammaglobulinemia, 180t
Hyperkeratosis, 173
Hyperplasia, reticuloendothelial system (RES) hyperplasia, 227
Hyperpyrexia, 2
Hypochlorhydric states, associated organisms, 267t
Hypogammaglobulinemia, 180t
Hypoparathyroidism, associated organisms, 267t

Immunoglobulin deficiency, 262
Immunosuppressed patients
and FUO, 8
See also Compromised host
Immunosuppressive drugs, 262
Impetigo, 232
Infectious hepatitis, and polyarthritis, 175, 186t
Infectious mononucleosis, 148, 229–230, 236, 241t, 253t
causes of mono syndrome, 216
and jaundice, 207t
and splenomegaly, 214, 216, 222t
See also Epstein-Barr virus (EBV)
Infective endocarditis, and splenomegaly, 224–225t
Inflammatory bowel disease, 180t
Influenza, and viral pneumonia, 24
Influenza vaccine, 271
INH, and CSF pleocytosis, 73t
Interferon alpha, 1
Interleukin 1, 1
Intermittent fever, 2
Intrathecal medication, and CSF pleocytosis, 73t

Intravenous pyelogram (IVP), 95
Iron hematoxylin, 122
Isoniazid, 7
Isoniazid prophylaxis, for pneumonia, 33–34t
Isospora, 122, 128t
Itraconazole, for pneumonia, 41t, 42t, 43t

Janeway spots, 5
Jaundice
anti-infective agents that cause, 195, 197
C. perfringens, 197–198, 203t
causes of, 196t
cholangitis, 205t
cholecystitis, 198–199, 204t
drugs that cause, 197
gonococcal perihepatitis, 199, 205–206t
hemolysis associated with infection, 196t, 197–198
hepatic jaundice associated with infection, 196t, 200–202
hyperbilirubinemia, 195
infectious mononucleosis, 207t
leptospirosis, 207–208t
liver abscess-amebic, 211t
liver abscess-pyogenic, 209–210t
posthepatic jaundice associated with infection, 196t, 198–200
pancreatitis, 199, 203–204t
pylephlebitis, 209t
Q fever, 201, 208t
recommended reading, 316
syphilitic hepatitis, 198, 200, 208t
viral hepatitis, 206t
Juvenile rheumatoid arthritis, 3, 192–193t

K. pneumoniae, 201
Kala-azar fever, 3, 219
Kaposi's sarcoma, 285, 289t

Kawasaki disease, 147, 158–159t, 231–232
Keratoderma blennorrhagica, 173
Ketoconazole, 283
Kidney infections
  acute pyelonephritis, 96, 108t, 111t
  perinephric abscess, 97, 110t
  renal abscess, 96–97, 109t
Kinin activation, 263
Klebsiella, and cystitis, 94
Klebsiella pneumonia, 18–19, 30t, 59

L. monocytogenes, CSF cell count, 59–60
Laboratory diagnosis, for bacterial pneumonia, 21–24
Laboratory procedures, patient with FUO, 6, 9–11t
Laparoscopy, 7, 10t
Lead encephalopathy, and CSF pleocytosis, 73t
Legionellosis
  and pneumonia, 14t, 20–21, 35t
  transmission of, 310t
Leishmaniasis, 146t
Leptospiral meningitis, 69, 80–81t
Leptospirosis, 3, 200
  and jaundice, 207–208t
  and pneumonia, 26
  transmission of, 310t
Leukemia, 8, 180t, 218t
  associated organisms, 267t
Leukocyte esterate dipstick, 89
Leukocyte stimulating factors, 270
Leukocytosis, 302
Leukoencephalopathy, and AIDS, 294t
LGV. *See* Lymphogranuloma venereum (LGV)
Listeria, transmission of, 310t
Listeria meningitis, 59–60, 76–77t
Liver, biopsy, 6, 9t
Lumbar puncture (LP), 6
  contraindication to, 65
  diagnosis of CNS infection, 54

Lung scan, 10t
Lyme disease, 69, 80–81t, 147
  and polyarthritis, 178, 188t
  rash, 143, 158–159t
  transmission of, 310t
Lymphadenopathy
  categories of, 227, 228t
  generalized adenopathy, 236–238
  local adenopathy
    axillary or epitrochlear adenopathy
      herpes zoster infection, 234, 249t
      herpetic whitlow, 234, 235, 250t
      sporotrichosis, 234, 249t
    cervical adenitis, 229–232
      MLNS (Kawasaki disease), 231–232
      mycobacterial adenitis, 230–231
      pharyngitis, 229–230
    inguinal adenopathy, caused by STDs, 235–236
    occipital adenopathy, 232
    peripheral axillary, epitrochlear, and inguinal adenopathy, 232–235
  lymph node biopsy, 229
  noninfectious causes of, 239t
  recommended reading, 316–317
  generalized lymphadenopathy
    brucellosis, 237, 258t
    CMV, 236, 254t
    dengue fever, 236–237, 255t
    histoplasmosis, 237–238, 259t
    HIV, 237, 259t
    infectious mononucleosis, 236, 253t
    measles, 236, 255t
    rubella, 236–237, 253t
    secondary syphilis, 238, 259t
    toxoplasmosis, 237, 256t

Lymphadenopathy
  selected etiologies—*continued*
    tuberculosis, 238, 258t
    tularemia, 236, 257t
  inguinal adenopathy
    chancroid, 235, 251t
    granuloma inguinale, 236, 252t
    herpes simplex, 236, 252t
    LGV, 235–236, 250–251t
    primary syphilis, 235, 250t
  MLNS (Kawasaki disease), 231–232, 245t
  mycobacterial adenitis, 230–231, 244t
  occipital adenopathy
    nonspecific scalp infection, 232, 245t
    rubella, 232, 245t
  peripheral adenopathy
    bacterial adenitis, 232–233, 246t
    cat-scratch disease, 233, 246–247t
    plague, 233–234, 248t
    rat-bite fever, 234, 248t
    tularemia, 233, 247t
  pharyngitis
    A. hemolyticum, 230, 243t
    diphtheria, 231, 242t
    fusospirochetal infection, 231, 243t
    gonococcus, 230, 243t
    Group A streptococcal, 229, 240–241t
    infectious mononucleosis, 229–230, 241t
    viral, 229, 240t
    Yersinia, 230, 243t
Lymphangitis, 233
Lymphocytic choriomeningitis (LCM), 3, 71, 72
  transmission of, 310t
Lymphocytosis, 303

Lymphogranuloma venereum (LGV), 227, 235–236, 250–251t
  arthritis, 179, 189t
Lymphoma, 180t, 218t
  associated organisms, 267t

M. Avium complex (MAC), 230
  and AIDS, 280, 283, 288t, 298t
M. hemophilum, 146t
M. marinum, 146t
M. scrofulaceum, 230
M. tuberculosis, 21, 33–34t, 123, 230–231, 244t
  and AIDS, 283, 288t
  and prostatitis, 93
M. ulcerans, 146t
Malaria, 69–70, 80–81t
  and jaundice, 197
  and pneumonia, 14t
  and splenomegaly, 217, 221t
  transmission of, 311t
Marantic endocarditis, 174
Mastoiditis, CSF response, 67
Mayaro virus, 177
Measles, 236, 255t
  encephalopathies and, 68
Mebendazole, 44t, 45t
Melioidosis, 146t
  and pneumonia, 14t
  transmission of, 311t
Meningismus fever, 66
Meningitis
  amebic meningitis, 62, 76–77t
  "aseptic" meningitis, 64
  bacterial meningitis
    age-related pathogens, 57
    diagnostic studies to detect etiology of, 60, 61t
  fungal meningitis, 64, 76–77t
  H. influenzae meningitis, 59
  herpes simplex types 1 & 2, meningoencephalitis, 70–71, 82–83t
  Leptospiral meningitis, 69, 80–81t

Lyme disease, 68–69, 80–81t
malaria, 69–70, 80–81t
meningococcal and
    meningococcemia, 58
partially treated bacterial
    meningitis, 65, 76–77t
pneumococcal, 57–58
other causes of, 59–60
syphilitic meningitis, 68–69,
    78–79t
toxoplasmosis, 70, 80–81t
trichinosis, 70, 80–81t
tuberculosis meningitis, 62–63,
    76–77t
Meningococcal endocarditis, 3
Meningococcemia, 5
    polyarthritis, 173, 182t
    rash, 137–138, 150–151t
Meningoencephalitis, and AIDS,
    285–286, 293–294t
Mesenteric adenitis, 121
Metastatic neoplasm, 218t
Metronidazole
    and CSF pleocytosis, 73t
    for pneumonia, 31t, 44t
Microsporidia, 128t
Miliary tuberculosis, 33–34t, 238
    and splenomegaly, 220t
Mitral regurgitation, 174
MLNS. *See* Mucocutaneous lymph
    node syndrome (MLNS)
Molecular biologic techniques, for
    pneumonia diagnosis, 23
Mollaret's syndrome, and CSF
    pleocytosis, 84–85t73t
Mollusium contagiosum, and AIDS,
    296t
Monoarthritis
    bacterial etiology, 163–165, 168t
    causes of, 164t
    infectious, 168–169t
    less common etiologies, 166
    noninfectious, 166, 167t
    recommended reading, 315
    septic arthritis, 163
    tuberculosis arthritis, 165–166,
    168t
Monocytosis, 303

Moraxella catarrhalis, 19
MRI, 6, 9t
Mucocutaneous lymph node
    syndrome (MLNS), 147,
    231–232, 245t
Multiple myeloma, associated
    organisms, 268t
Mumps
    and CSF levels, 71
    encephalopathies and, 68
    and polyarthritis, 176, 185t
Murine typhus, transmission of,
    311t
Mushroom poisoning, and diarrhea,
    124
Mycobacterial infection, 122
    and adenitis, 230–231, 244t
    and AIDS, 296t
    and arthritis, 166
Mycoplasma infection
    and jaundice, 198
    rash, 143, 147, 156–157t
Mycoplasmal pneumonia
    (*Mycoplasma pneumoniae*),
    15–16, 71, 78–79t
Myelography, and CSF pleocytosis,
    73t
Myelophthisic anemia, 218t
Myocarditis, 299t
Myopericardial syndromes, 72
Myositis, and AIDS, 299t

N. gonorrhoeae, 90
Naegleria fowleri, causing
    meningoencephalitis, 62
Nafcillin, for pneumonia, 29t
Naprosen therapy, for FUO, 8
Nasopharyngeal suction, for
    pneumonia diagnosis, 23
Neisserial infections, disseminated,
    262–263
Neisserias catarrhalis, 19
    causing petechiae, 137
Nematodes, and pneumonia, 14t
Neonatal meningitis, 59

Neonates
  febrile response to infection, 2
  jaundice in, 201
Neoplasm, 180t, 218t
Nephrotic syndrome, associated
    organisms, 268t
Neuropathic joints, 178
Neutropenia, associated organisms,
    268t
Neutrophil activation, 263
Neutrophil transfusions, 270
Nicolsky's sign, 147
Nitrite reduction test, 89
Nocardia, and pneumonia, 14t
Nocardiosis, 146t, 234
Non-gonococcal urethritis (NGU),
    92, 102t
Non-Hodgkin's lymphoma, and
    AIDS, 285, 289t
Noninfectious polyarthritis, 180t
Nonspecific urethritis (NSU), 102t
Nonsteroidal antiinflammatory
    drugs (NSAIDS), and CSF
    pleocytosis, 73t
Nonthrombocytopenic purpura, 136
Nuclear stains, 122

Ockelbo virus, 177
Ofloxacin, for pneumonia, 34t
OKT$_3$, and CSF pleocytosis, 73t
O'nyong-nyong fever, 177
Ophthalmologic complications,
    AIDS, 287, 300t
Opportunistic pathogens, 8
  and the compromised host,
      265–266
    associated with humoral or T-
        cell defects, 266t
    associated with particular
        medical conditions,
        267–268t
Opsonins, 262, 263
Optic neuritis, and AIDS, 300t
Orchitis, and prostatitis, 93
Osler's nodes, 5
"Osler's triad," 67

Osteoarthritis, 169t
Osteochondritis, causing
    monoarthritis, 167t
Osteomyelitis, CSF response, 67,
    78–79t
Otitis, CSF response, 67, 78–79t

P. aeruginosa, 19, 30–31t, 121, 139
  infection, as complication of LPs,
      59
Palindromic rheumatism, 167t,
    180t
Pancreatitis, 283
  and jaundice, 199, 203–204t
Pancytopenia, 306
Papillary necrosis, 97–98, 108–109t
Parainfluenza, and viral
    pneumonia, 24
Parameningeal infections, 65–68,
    78–79t
Parasites
  associated with humoral or T-cell
      defects, 266t
  and pneumonia, 14t, 15t
Parasitic causes of diarrheal
    diseases, 121–122
  amebiasis, 122–123, 132t
  giardiasis, 123, 128t
Paroxysmal cold hemoglobinuria,
    198
Paroxysmal nocturnal
    hemoglobinuria (PNH),
    198
Parvovirus, 116t, 116–117
  and polyarthritis, 175–176, 186t
Parvovirus B19, 306
Pastia's lines, 145
Pediculosis capitis, 232
Penicillin, 60
Penicillin G, 69
  for pneumonia, 29t, 36t
Periodic acid stain (PAS), 229
Peripheral neuropathy, and AIDS,
    286, 295t
Phagocytosis, 262–263
Pharyngeal pseudomembrane,
    causes of, 231

Pharyngitis, 229–230
  A. hemolyticum, 230, 243t
  diphtheria, 231, 242t
  fusospirochetal infection, 231, 243t
  gonococcus, 230, 243t
  Group A streptococcal, 229, 240–241t
  infectious mononucleosis, 229–230, 241t
  viral, 229, 240t
  Yersinia, 230, 243t
Pharyngotonsillitis, 280
Phycomycetes, and pneumonia in the compromised host, 15t, 26–27, 48t
PIE syndrome, 51t
Pigmented villonodular synovitis, causing monoarthritis, 167t
Piperacillin, for pneumonia, 30t, 31t
Piperazine, for pneumonia, 44t
Plague, 233–234, 248t
  and pneumonia, 14t, 26
  transmission of, 311t
Platelets, changes in
  thrombocytopenia, 304–305
  thrombocytosis, 305
Pleurodynia, 72
Pneumococcal meningitis, 57–58
Pneumococcal pneumonia, 17, 28t
Pneumococcal vaccine, 271
Pneumococci, and septic arthritis in children, 163
Pneumocystic carinii, 8, 26, 48t, 280, 286
Pneumonitis
  anaerobic pneumonia, 19–20, 31–32t
  bacterial pneumonia, 16
  causes of, 13, 15–15t, 16
    age-related, 15
  chlamydia pneumoniae, 21, 35t
  in the compromised host, 26–27, 46–48t
  epidemiologic clues to etiology, 26
  gram-negative bacilli, 18, 30t
  haemophilus pneumonia, 20, 29t
  Klebsiella pneumonia, 18–19, 30t
  laboratory diagnosis, bacterial pneumonia, 21–24
  Legionnaire's disease, 20–21, 35t
  mycoplasmal pneumonia, 15–16
  noninfectious causes of, 27, 27t
  pneumococcal pneumonia, 17, 28t
  pseudomonas pneumonia, 19, 30–31t
  pulmonary syndromes confused with, 50–51t
  recommended reading, 313
  staphylococcal and gram-negative rod pneumonia, 17, 29t
  staphylococcal pneumonia, 17–18, 29t
  treatment of, 23–24, 28–51t
  tuberculosis, 21, 33–34t
  viral pneumonias, 24–25, 28t
Poliomyelitis, 72
Polyarthritis, 5
  acute rheumatic fever, 175, 191t
  arbovirus arthritis, 177
  bacterial endocarditis, 174, 183–184t
  causes of, 172t
  coccidioidomycosis, 176–177, 187t
  gonococcal arthritis, 171–173, 181t
  HIV infection, 176, 186t
  infectious hepatitis, 175, 186t
  juvenile rheumatoid arthritis, 193–194t
  Lyme disease, 178, 188t
  lymphogranuloma venereum arthritis, 179, 189t
  meningococcemia, 173, 182t
  noninfectious polyarthritis, 180t
  parvovirus, 175–176, 186t
  rash, 138
  rat-bite fever, 178, 184t, 188t
  reactive arthritis, 174
  recommended reading, 315–316
  Reiter's syndrome, 173–174, 190t

Polyarthritis—*continued*
  rheumatoid arthritis, 193t
  rubella and mumps, 176, 185t
  sarcoidosis, 177, 192t
  serum sickness, 192t
  SLE, 175, 190–191t
  syphilitic arthritis, 178, 187t
  Whipple's disease, 179, 190t
Polycythemia vera, 218t
Polymerase chain reaction (PCR), 60, 61t
  for pneumonia diagnosis, 23
Polymorphonuclear leukocytes (PMLs), 1
  abnormalities of PML function, 263, 264–265t
Polymyalgia rheumatica, 5
Portal vein obstruction, 218t
Postperfusion syndrome, 236
Pregnancy, symptomatic UTI and, 98
Proctitis, 120
Prostatitis
  acute form, 93, 104t
  chronic form, 93–94, 105t
  nonbacterial, 94, 105t
  prostatic abscess, 93, 106t
  prostatodynia, 94
Prosthetic heart valves, 224–225t
Proteus
  and cystitis, 94
  and pneumonia, 18
Protozoal diarrhea, 122, 128t
Pseudoappendicitis, 121
  in AIDS, 285
Pseudogout, 167t, 169t, 179t
Pseudomembranous colitis, 120
Pseudomonads
  bacteremia, 139
  and cystitis, 94
  and meningitis, 59
  and pneumonia, 18, 19, 30–31t
  and septicemia, 139
Psittacosis
  and pneumonia, 14t, 26
  rash, 143

  and splenomegaly, 216–217, 225t
  transmission of, 311t
"Psychogenic fever," 7
Pulmonary edema, 25
Pulmonary embolism, 50t, 66
Pulmonary infiltrate, in the compromised host, 268
Pulmonary syndromes, in AIDS, 286–287, 298–299t
Purpura fulminans, 137
Purulent meningitis, 67
Pyelonephritis, 96, 108t, 111t
Pylephlebitis, 201
  and jaundice, 209t
Pyrimethamine, for pneumonia, 49t
Pyrimethamine-sulfadiazine, 283
Pyrogens, endogenous, 1
Pyuria. *See* Urinary tract infection (UTI)

Q fever, 3
  and jaundice, 201, 208t
  and pneumonia, 14t, 26
  transmission of, 311t
Quellung reaction, 60, 61t
Quinolone
  for pneumonia, 38t
  for prostatitis, 100

R. conorii, rash, 142, 144, 156–157t
R. prowazekii, 142
Rabies, transmission of, 311t
Radiculitis, 69
Rash
  cellulitis-etiology, 145t
  maculopapular rashes
    Lyme disease, 143, 158–159t
    mycoplasma infection, 143, 156–157t
    psittacosis, 143
    rickettsial diseases, 142, 154–155t
    secondary syphilis, 141–142, 154–155t
    typhoid fever, 142–143, 156–157t

INDEX

noninfectious causes of rash, 149t
petechial and purpuric rashes
  bacterial endocarditis, 137, 150–151t
  disseminated intravascular coagulation (DIC), 136–137, 156–157t
  gonococcemia, 138, 152–153t
  meningococcemia, 137–138, 150–151t
  nonthrombocytopenic purpura, 136
  other bacteremias, 139, 152–153t
  rat-bite fevers, 141, 154–155t
  rickettsial infections, 139–140, 154–155t
and pneumonia, 26
recommended reading, 315
types of
  no specific treatment for, 135t
  specific treatment for, 134t
  ulcerating lesions, 146t
  urticarial rash, 147
    drug reactions, 147–148
  vesicular/bullous or pustular rash, 144, 160–161t
    diffuse erythemas, 144–145, 147, 158–159t
Rat flea, 142
Rat-bite fever, 234, 248t
and polyarthritis, 178, 184t, 188t
rash, 141, 154–155t
transmission of, 311t
Reactive arthritis, and Reiter's syndrome, 174
Red blood cells (RBCs), changes in, 305–306
Reiter's syndrome, and polyarthritis, 173–174, 190t
Relapsing fever, 2, 3
Remittent fever, 2
Respiratory syncytial virus (RSV), 24, 25
Reticuloendothelial hyperplasia, 214

Reticuloendothelial system (RES) hyperplasia, 227
Retinitis, and AIDS, 300t
Rheumatic fever, 5
and polyarthritis, 175, 191t
Rheumatoid arthritis, 5, 167t, 169t, 193t
Rickettsial infections/diseases, 68, 225t
and pneumonia, 26
rash, 139–140, 142, 154–155t
transmission of, 311t
Rifampin, 7, 283
  for pneumonia, 38t
Ringworm, 232
Rochalimaea (Bartorella) *henselae*, 233
Rocky Mountain spotted fever (RMSF), 68, 80–81t
rash, 139–140, 142, 154–155t
and splenomegaly, 216, 225t
transmission of, 309t, 311t
"Rose spots"
  and pneumonia, 26
  and typhoid fever, 143, 156–157t
Roseola infantum, 237
Ross River virus, 177
Roth spots, 5, 137, 174
Rotoviruses, 116t, 116–117
Rubella, 200, 232, 236–237, 245t, 253t
  and polyarthritis, 176, 185t
  rash, 140
Rubeola, 232, 245t
  rash, 140
  and viral pneumonia, 24

S. aureus, 67, 116t, 127t, 131t, 214, 224t
  and septic arthritis in children, 163
S. minus, 234
S. typhi, 120, 121, 201, 223t
S. viridans bacteremia, 147
Salicylates, as cause of chills, 2–3

INDEX

Salmonella, 201
  and Reiter's syndrome, 174
Salmonellosis, 5
  and diarrhea, 119, 129t
  and pneumonia, 14t
  transmission of, 312t
Sarcoid, and CSF pleocytosis, 73t, 84–85t
Sarcoidosis, 180t, 218t
  and polyarthritis, 177, 192t
SBE. *See* Subacute bacterial endocarditis (SBE)
Scabies, and AIDS, 297t
Scalp infections, 232, 245t
Scarlet fever, 144, 145
  encephalopathies and, 68
Schistosoma cutis, 146t
Schistosomiasis, 219
Sedimentation rate (ESR), 306
Seizure activity, and CSF pleocytosis, 73t, 84–85t
Sepsis, nonspecific signs of, 8
Septic arthritis, in children, 163
Septic monoarthritis, 163, 165
Septicemia, 25, 201, 202
Serology tests, 11t
Serotype 0157:H7, 118
Serum sickness, 180t
  and polyarthritis, 192t
"Shanghai Fever," 121, 139
Shellfish, contaminated, 120
Shigella, and Reiter's syndrome, 173
Shigellosis
  and diarrhea, 113, 118–119, 129t
  transmission of, 312t
Shingles, and AIDS, 296t
Sickle cell anemia, 198, 262
  associated organisms, 268t
Sindbis virus, 177
Sinusitis, 66
  and AIDS, 287, 300t
  CSF response, 67, 78–79t
SLE. *See* Systemic lupus erythematosus (SLE)
Smears, techniques for, petechiae, 138

S/P intestinal bypass, 180t
Specimen collecting, for UTIs, 88
Spinal anesthesia, and CSF pleocytosis, 73t
Spirillum minus, 178
  rash, 141
  transmission of, 311t
Spirillum moniliformis,
  transmission of, 311t
Splenectomy, associated organisms, 268t
Splenic vein obstruction, 218t
Splenomegaly, 5, 174, 200
  acute: infectious causes of, 215t
    bacteremia, 214
    malaria, 217
    psittacosis, 216–217
    RMSF, 216
    viremia, 214, 216
  "acute splenic tumor," 214
  noninfectious causes of, 218t, 219
  and pneumonia, 26
  rare causes of, 219
  recommended reading, 316
  selected etiologies
    disseminated histoplasmosis, 220–221t
    infectious mononucleosis-EBV, 222t
    infective endocarditis, 224–225t
    malaria, 221t
    miliary tuberculosis, 220t
    psittacosis, 225t
    RMSF, 225t
    typhoid fever, 223–224t
  spleen, function of, 213
  subacute or chronic causes of
    disseminated histoplasmosis, 219
    disseminated tuberculosis, 218–219
    SBE, 217–218
Splinter hemorrhages, 5
Sporotrichosis, 146t, 234, 249t
Sporotrichum schenkii, 234, 249t
Sputum smear, for pneumonia diagnosis, 22

INDEX   337

Staph scalded skin syndrome (SSSS), 145
Staphylococcal and gram-negative rod pneumonia, 17, 29t
Staphylococcal enterocolitis, and diarrhea, 120
Staphylococcal food poisoning, and diarrhea, 117
Staphylococcal pneumonia, 17–18, 29t
Staphylococcemia, rash, 139, 144
Stavudine (d4T), 283
"Strawberry tongue," 145
Streptobacillus moniliformis, 178, 234
   rash, 141
Streptococcal meningitis, 59
Streptococcal pyrogenic exotoxins, 145, 160–161t
Streptococcemia, rash, 139
Streptococcus pneumoniae, 201, 214
Streptococcus pyogenes, 229
Streptomycin, 7, 37t
Strongyloides, and pneumonia in the compromised host, 15t
Strongyloidiasis, 122
Subacute bacterial endocarditis (SBE), 5, 9t
   and splenomegaly, 217–218
Sulfonamides
   and CSF pleocytosis, 73t
   for pneumonia, 45t
Surgery, GI, associated organisms, 267t
Surveillance Case definition, AIDS, 281, 282t
Sustained fever, 2
Syphilis, 146t
   and AIDS, 294t
   primary, 235, 250t
   rash, 141–142, 154–155t
   secondary, 238, 259t
Syphilitic arthritis, 178, 187t
Syphilitic hepatitis, and jaundice, 198, 200, 208t
Syphilitic meningitis, 68–69, 78–79t

Systemic lupus erythematosus (SLE), 5, 218t, 238, 262
   and CSF findings, 84–85t
   and polyarthritis, 175, 191–192t

T. pallidum, 123
Taenia solium/saginata, transmission of, 312t
Tazobactam, for pneumonia, 31t
Temperature, body. *See* Fever
Tenosynovitis, 164
   and arthritis, 173
   rash, 138
Tetracycline, 37t, 69
Therapeutic drug trials, for cause of FUO, 7
Thiabendazole, for pneumonia, 45t
Thrombocytopenia, 304–305
Thrombocytosis, 305
Thrombophlebitis, cerebral, 66, 78–79t
Thrombotic thrombocytopenic purpura, 218t
Ticarcillin-clavulanate, for pneumonia, 31t
Tick exposure, 68 TMP-SMX, 283
   for prostatitis, 100
TMP-SMZ
   and CSF pleocytosis, 73t
Tobramycin, for pneumonia, 30t
Toxic epidermal necrolysis (TEN), 147
Toxic shock syndrome, 145
Toxin-induced gastroenteritis, 124, 125t
Toxoplasma, 200
   and pneumonia, 26
   in the compromised host, 15t
Toxoplasmosis, 5, 70, 80–81t, 237, 256t
   and AIDS, 293t
   transmission of, 312t
Transmission of infectious disease, other than person-to-person spread, 307, 308–312t

338 INDEX

Transplant recipient, receiving immunosuppressives, associated organisms, 268t
Transtracheal aspiration, for pneumonia diagnosis, 23
Traube's space, 213
Trauma, causing monoarthritis, 167t, 169t
Travel, international, as source of FUO, 7
Traveler's diarrhea, 122
Trichinosis, 70, 80–81t
　transmission of, 312t
Trichomonal urethritis, 92, 103t
Trichrome stain, 122
Trimethoprim, and CSF pleocytosis, 73t
Trimethoprimsulfamethoxazole, for pneumonia, 48t
Tropheryma whippeli, 179
Trophozoites, 121
TSST-1 toxin, 145
Tuberculosis, 146t, 238, 258t
　and AIDS, 293t, 298t
　antituberculosis therapy, 7
　arthritis, 164t, 165–166, 168t
　and cystitis, 95
　disseminated, and splenomegaly, 218–219
　meningitis, 62–63, 76–77t
　and pneumonia, 21, 33–34t
　and pyelonephritis, 96
　search for, 9t
Tularemia, 146t, 233, 236, 247t, 257t
　and pneumonia, 14t, 26
　transmission of, 312t
Tumor (s)
　and AIDS, 289t
　causing monoarthritis, 167t
　and CSF pleocytosis, 73t, 84–85t
　occult, search for, 5–6, 10t
Tumor necrosis factor, 1
Typhoid fever, 3
　and diarrhea, 132t
　and pneumonia, 14t, 26
　rash, 142–143, 156–157t
　and splenomegaly, 223–224t
Typhus
　murine, 142, 156–157t
　rash, 139–140
　transmission of, 312t

Ulcerating lesions, 146t
Ulcerative colitis, 120, 121
Ureaplasma, and Reiter's syndrome, 173
Ureaplasma urealyticum, 92
Urethritis, 92, 102–103t
Urinary tract infection (UTI)
　categories of, 91t
　cystitis, 94–95, 106–107t, 110–111t
　GU tuberculosis, 95, 112t
　kidney infections
　　acute pyelonephritis, 96, 108t, 111t
　　perinephric abscess, 97, 110t
　　renal abscess, 96–97, 109t
　laboratory tests for, 88–90
　management of, 99–101
　other infections
　　abscesses outside the GU tract, 98
　　asymptomatic bacteriuria, 98–99
　　papillary necrosis, 97–98, 108–109t
　prostatitis
　　acute form, 93, 104t
　　chronic form, 93–94, 105t
　　nonbacterial, 94, 105t
　　prostatic abscess, 93, 106t
　　prostatodynia, 94
　recommended reading, 314
　recurrent infection, 100
　specimen collecting, 88
　suprapubic puncture, 89
　symptomatology, 87–88
　upper *vs.* lower tract infection, distinguishing between, 89–90

urethral catheterization, 89
urethritis, 92, 102–103t
Urine specimen collecting, for UTIs, 88
Urticarial rash, 147

V. cholerae, 116t, 117
Vaccination
　encephalopathies and, 68
　and immunocompromised patients, 271
Vaginitis, 90
Vaginosis, 90
Vancomycin, 29t, 58
Varicella, and viral pneumonia, 24, 25
Varicella-zoster, 144
　and AIDS, 299t
　CSF findings, 71, 82–83t
　and pneumonia in the compromised host, 14t
Vasculitis, and CSF pleocytosis, 73t
Vibrio parahaemolyticus, and diarrhea, 120–121, 131t
Vibrio vulnificus, skin lesions, 144, 160–161t
Viral gastroenteritis, cause of diarrheal disease, 116–117, 126t
Viral hepatitis, and jaundice, 206t
Viral infections, rash from, 140
Viral meningoencephalitis, 71, 72, 82–83t
Viral neutralization, 263
Viral pneumonia, 24–25, 28t
　in the compromised host, 14t
Viremia, and splenomegaly, 214, 216
Viruses, associated with humoral or T-cell defects, 266t

Weil-Felix reaction, 201
Whipple's disease, and polyarthritis, 179, 190t
White blood count (WBC)
　increased, 301–302
　normal or slightly depressed, 302
　severely depressed, 302

Yellow fever, transmission of, 312t
Yersinia
　and pharyngitis, 230, 243t
　and Reiter's syndrome, 173
Yersinia enterocolitica infection, and diarrhea, 119, 129t
Yersinia pestis, and pneumonia, 26, 27t

Zalcitabine (ddC), 283
ZDV, 283
Zidovudine, 283
Ziehl-Neelsen stain, 229
Zoster immune globulin (ZIG), 144, 271